BIOLOGICAL
CARCINOGENESIS

edited by

Marvin A. Rich and Philip Furmanski
AMC Cancer Research Center and Hospital
Lakewood, Colorado

MARCEL DEKKER, INC.   New York and Basel

Library of Congress Cataloging in Publication Data
Main entry under title:

Biological carcinogenesis.

    Includes bibliographical references and index.
    1. Carcinogenesis. I. Rich, Marvin A. II. Furmanski,
Philip, [date].   [DNLM: 1. Carcinogens--Congresses.
2. Neoplasms--Etiology--Congresses. QZ 202 B6155 1980]
RC268.5.B56   616.99'4071   82-4996
ISBN 0-8247-1635-3   AACR2

MARCEL DEKKER, INC.
270 Madison Avenue, New York, New York 10016

Current printing (last digit):
10 9 8 7 6 5 4 3 2 1

PRINTED IN THE UNITED STATES OF AMERICA

PREFACE

Neoplastic transformation can be induced by biological, chemical and physical agents. Are the mechanisms underlying carcinogenesis by these classes of agents the same, or are they as diverse as their properties are distinctive? Are the interactions which occur between the classes of carcinogens important factors in cancer causation and progression? And finally, can conceptual and technological advances made for one type of carcinogen be brought to bear on the resolution of the mechanistic mysteries which surround the others?

To address these questions, scientists in the forefront of viral, chemical and physical carcinogenesis, including those few individuals engaged in studies involving *combined modalities* of carcinogenesis, gathered in Detroit for a workshop on Biological Carcinogenesis, organized and supported by the Michigan Cancer Foundation and the National Cancer Institute.

In this volume, which originated from the Workshop presentations and discussions, the authors have identified the general principles which govern carcinogenesis by each of the major classes of carcinogens and determined to what extent these principles are applicable to the carcinogenic process induced by other classes of agents. There is described, in addition, current knowledge on the interaction of carcinogens and the identification of biological systems where viral, chemical, and physical carcinogens are demonstrably interactive and thus, provide effective systems for the further study of this phenomenon.

To date, our mechanistic understanding of the carcinogenic process is painfully sparse and can ill afford less than optimum communication between those who study its diverse parts. It was

the aim of this workshop, and of this volume, to encourage and
stimulate the full use of knowledge developed in one sphere of
carcinogenic research by investigators in the others.

The editors and authors wish to thank the members of the
Organizing Committee, Dr. Leila Diamond, Dr. Charles M. King, Dr.
Charles M. McGrath and Dr. Louis R. Sibal for their enthusiastic
participation in the development of the workshop, and the Michigan
Cancer Foundation and the Division of Cancer Cause and Prevention
of the National Cancer Institute of the United States for their
support of the workshop.

Marvin A. Rich

Philip Furmanski

CONTENTS

CONTRIBUTORS

LARRY O. ARTHUR   *Biological Carcinogenesis Program, Frederick Cancer Research Center, Frederick, Maryland*

LAURE AURELIAN   *Department of Biochemistry and Biophysics, Division of Comparative Medicine, The Johns Hopkins Medical Institutions, Baltimore, Maryland*

P. A. BENTVELZEN   *Radiobiological Institute TNO, Rijswijk, The Netherlands*

JANET S. BUTEL   *Department of Virology and Epidemiology, Baylor College of Medicine, Houston, Texas*

TIMOTHY H. CARTER   *Department of Biological Sciences, St. John's University, Jamaica, New York*

ALAIN DECLEVE*   *Cancer Biology Research Laboratory, Department of Radiology, Stanford University School of Medicine, Stanford, California*

JOSEPH E. DE LARCO   *Laboratory of Viral Carcinogenesis, National Cancer Institute, Frederick Cancer Research Center, Frederick, Maryland*

SANDRA K. DUSING-SWARTZ   *Department of Cell Biology, Baylor College of Medicine, Houston, Texas*

PAUL B. FISHER   *Department of Microbiology, Cancer Center/ Institute of Cancer Research, College of Physicians and Surgeons, Columbia University, New York, New York*

PHILIP FURMANSKI†   *Department of Biology, Michigan Cancer Foundation, Detroit, Michigan*

*Current Affiliation: Risk Management Division, Stanford University School of Medicine, Stanford, California
†Current Affiliation: AMC Cancer Research Center and Hospital, Lakewood, Colorado

ROBERT C. GALLO   *Laboratory of Tumor Cell Biology, National Cancer Institute, National Institutes of Health, Bethesda, Maryland*

RAYMOND V. GILDEN   *Biological Carcinogenesis Program, Frederick Cancer Research Center, Frederick, Maryland*

NEIL I. GOLDSTEIN   *Monell Chemical Senses Center, Philadelphia, Pennsylvania*

PHILIP L. GROVER   *Chester Beatty Research Institute, Institute of Cancer Research, Royal Cancer Hospital, London, United Kingdom*

RUSSELL EARL HAND, JR.   *Biology Division, Oak Ridge National Laboratory, Oak Ridge, Tennessee*

DAVID K. HOWARD   *Life Sciences Division, Meloy Laboratories, Inc., Springfield, Virginia*

ELIEZER HUBERMAN   *Toxicology and Carcinogenesis Program, Biology Division, Oak Ridge National Laboratory, Oak Ridge, Tennessee*

CANDACE S. JOHNSON   *Department of Biology, Michigan Cancer Foundation, Detroit, Michigan*

CAROL A. JONES   *Toxicology and Carcinogenesis Program, Biology Division, Oak Ridge National Laboratory, Oak Ridge, Tennessee*

RICHARD F. JONES   *Department of Tumor Biology, Michigan Cancer Foundation, Detroit, Michigan*

HENRY S. KAPLAN   *Cancer Biology Research Laboratory, Department of Radiology, Stanford University School of Medicine, Stanford, California*

JAMES O. KIGGANS, JR.   *Biology Division, Oak Ridge National Laboratory, Oak Ridge, Tennessee*

V. KRUMP-KONVALINKOVA   *Radiobiological Institute TNO, Rijswijk, The Netherlands*

MIRIAM LIEBERMAN   *Cancer Biology Research Laboratory, Department of Radiology, Stanford University School of Medicine, Stanford, California*

RUEY-SHYAN LIOU   *Biology Division, Oak Ridge National Laboratory, Oak Ridge, Tennessee*

SIMONE MANTEUIL-BRUTLAG   *Cancer Biology Research Laboratory, Department of Radiology, Stanford University School of Medicine, Stanford, California*

MARK MAMRACK   *Biology Division, Oak Ridge National Laboratory, Oak Ridge, Tennessee*

MARK M. MANAK   *Departments of Biophysics and Comparative Medicine, The Johns Hopkins Medical Institutions, Baltimore, Maryland*

JOHN MARCELLETTI   *Department of Biology, Michigan Cancer Foundation, Detroit, Michigan*

CHARLES M. MCGRATH   *Department of Tumor Biology, Michigan Cancer Foundation, Detroit, Michigan*

DANIEL MEDINA   *Department of Cell Biology, Baylor College of Medicine, Houston, Texas*

JAMES A. OTTEN   *Biology Division, Oak Ridge National Laboratory, Oak Ridge, Tennessee*

MARVIN A. RICH*   *Michigan Cancer Foundation, Detroit, Michigan*

JEFFREY SCHLOM   *Laboratory of Cellular and Molecular Biology, National Cancer Institute, National Institutes of Health, Bethesda, Maryland*

THOMAS J. SLAGA   *Biology Division, Oak Ridge National Laboratory, Oak Ridge, Tennessee*

GILBERT H. SMITH   *Laboratory of Molecular Biology, National Cancer Institute, National Institutes of Health, Bethesda, Maryland*

SUSAN H. SOCHER   *Department of Cell Biology, Baylor College of Medicine, Houston, Texas*

HERBERT D. SOULE   *Department of Tumor Biology, Michigan Cancer Foundation, Detroit, Michigan*

RAYMOND W. TENNANT†   *Biology Division, Oak Ridge National Laboratory, Oak Ridge, Tennessee*

GEORGE J. TODARO   *Laboratory of Viral Carcinogenesis, National Cancer Institute, Frederick Cancer Research Center, Frederick, Maryland*

---

*Current Affiliation: AMC Cancer Research and Hospital, Lakewood, Colorado

†Current Affiliation: National Toxicology Program, National Institute of Environmental Health Sciences, Research Triangle Park, North Carolina

PAUL O. P. TS'O   *Division of Biophysics, School of Hygiene and Public Health, The Johns Hopkins Medical Institutions, Baltimore, Maryland*

D. W. VAN BEKKUM   *Radiobiological Institute TNO, Rijswijk, The Netherlands*

K. VAN DEN BERG   *Radiobiological Institute TNO, Rijswijk, The Netherlands*

TSE-WEI WANG   *Biology Division, Oak Ridge National Laboratory, and the University of Tennessee - Oak Ridge Graduate School of Biomedical Sciences, Oak Ridge, Tennessee*

I. BERNARD WEINSTEIN   *Department of Medicine/School of Public Health, and the Cancer Center/Institute for Cancer Research, College of Physicians and Surgeons, Columbia University, New York, New York*

WEN K. YANG   *Biology Division, Oak Ridge National Laboratory, Oak Ridge, Tennessee*

C. S. H. YOUNG   *Department of Microbiology, Institute for Cancer Research, College of Physicians and Surgeons, Columbia University, New York, New York*

HOWARD A. YOUNG   *Biological Carcinogenesis Program, Frederick Cancer Research Center, Frederick, Maryland*

MECHANISMS IN VIRAL CARCINOGENESIS

T-CELL GROWTH, T-CELL GROWTH FACTOR, T-CELL LEUKEMIAS AND LYMPHOMAS AND ISOLATION OF A NEW TYPE-C RETROVIRUS

Robert C. Gallo

Laboratory of Tumor Cell Biology
National Cancer Institute
National Institutes of Health
Bethesda, Maryland

SUMMARY

About 5 years ago we discovered a new system for the long term (continuous) growth of normal human T-cells. These include T cells with functional activities. The cells are mature T-lymphocytes positive in E-rosette assays and negative for the enzyme terminal deoxyribonucleotidyl transferase. The growth of these cells can far surpass the finite number of generations described for normal fibroblasts, and the cells remain normal in all criteria. Their growth is strictly dependent upon a factor we call T-cell growth factor (TCGF). TCGF is a small protein which binds to the surface only of antigen (or lectin) activated normal T-cells. Thus, TCGF appears to be the direct mitogen in the immune response of all T-cells. So called lymphocyte activation by antigen or lectin involves at least two important mechanisms. Some T-cells must recognize the antigen/lectin and form functional TCGF receptors; other T-cells release TCGF. The latter appears to be mediated by a prior interaction of lectin/antigen with macrophage which release lymphocyte activation factor which in turn stimulates the subset of T-cells to release TCGF. This event is normally transient because TCGF production is temporary. However, T-cell growth can be maintained in the laboratory by the periodic TCGF addition to the cultured cells. In contrast to normal T-cells, neoplastic T-cells obtained from patients with certain T-cell leukemias and lymphomas contain TCGF receptors and so respond directly to TCGF

3

(without requiring lectin or antigen activation). Several novel cell
lines from patients with cutaneous T-cell leukemias and lymphomas
(Sezary syndrome and mycosis fungoides) were established with TCGF.
In some cases the cells became independent of added TCGF but release
into the media their own TCGF.

Some of the T-cell cultures continuously release a new type-C
retrovirus. We call these viruses HTLV. They are unique (not related
to any animal viruses), and to date specific for these diseases.
Antibodies have been found in some human sera specifically reactive
with HTLV proteins, including the first patient from whom HTLV was
isolated. We propose that the abnormal proliferation characteristic
of leukemias and lymphomas of mature T-cells may involve abnormalities
in the TCGF T-cell interaction, and that HTLV may be involved in the
pathogenesis of these diseases.

INTRODUCTION

In this report I will summarize results of experiments from our labo-

ratory relating to control of proliferation of human T-cells both

normal and neoplastic. I will also describe the isolation of new

type-C retroviruses (RNA tumor viruses) from some of these cells and

why we believe these represent the first unambiguous isolation of

human retroviruses. Finally, I will formulate a working hypothesis

for the mechanism of transformation of these cells. The studies which

I will describe were in part carried out with my associates F. Ruscetti

Ruscetti, B. Poiesz, J. Mier, M. Reitz, and V. Kalyanaraman, and

portions of the work (those with clinical material from patient

C. R.) were performed in collaboration with J. Minna and his col-

leagues P. Bunn and A. Gazdar, all of the NCI-VA Clinical Medical

Oncology Branch in Washington, D.C.

The Continuous Growth of Normal
Functional Mature Human T-Cells

The ability to continuously grow normal human mature T-cells in liquid

suspension culture was achieved for the first time about 5 years ago

[1,2]. This has been widely confirmed and extended (see especially

work of K. Smith reviewed in [3], and is now almost routinely employed

in laboratories interested in T-cell biology. The system has extreme-

ly interesting and important features. First of all, despite long

term culture the cells remain normal in karyotype, have functional
(e.g., cytotoxic) activity, remain strictly dependent on a factor
termed T-cell growth factor (TCGF) for their growth (see below) and
do not produce tumors in nude mice. Second, the proliferation far
exceeds the finite generations number of cell divisions believed to
be the limit of proliferation of committed cells (Hayflick number),
indicating that mature T-cells have stem cell features. Third, the
cells can be cloned and used in numerous T-cell immunobiology experiments. Fourth, there is rationale for their clinical use. For example, by the combination of cloning techniques and the use of TCGF,
autologous cytotoxic T-cells for a tumor may be obtained in large
numbers and used in immunotherapy. In addition, the central role of
TCGF in T-cell proliferation makes it seem likely to us that immune
deficiencies due to diminished number of T-cells might be helped by
exogenous TCGF. Fifth, the availability of purified TCGF [4,5] and
its specific interaction with activated T-cells makes it possible to
study the interaction of a pure growth factor with a cloned population
of cells newly cultured from clinical specimens. Sixth, as discussed
later, this system recently led to the establishment of several new
kinds of neoplastic T-cell lines, and the available information suggests that T-cell-TCGF changes in the normal production and and/or
response to TCGF may be involved in the abnormal proliferation characteristic of T-cell leukemias and lymphomas. Some of the new cell
lines also led to the isolation of new kinds of type-C retroviruses
(see below).

Components of the System

Normal leukocytes are obtained from blood, bone marrow or spleen and
the mononuclear fraction separated from other leukocytes by nylon
column chromatography [6,7]. The cells are stimulated with lectin/
antigen (generally PHA). This leads to blastogenesis (activation)
of a subset of T-cells involving synthesis of DNA, some cell division
and if left as such termination of the culture. After the exposure
to the lectin/antigen TCGF is released into the media, probably by
a subset of T-cells different from those which respond to TCGF. Even-

tually, TCGF release ceases and the cultured cells terminate their
growth unless there is intervention. Apparently, macrophages mediate
the T-cell release of TCGF. After their interaction with lectin/
antigen the macrophages release a factor termed lymphocyte activating
factor which induces the T-cells to release TCGF. Thus, some adherent
cells are required. If exogenous TCGF is added every 3 to 4 days to
the cultured cells the T cells proliferate indefinitely (reviewed in
[8]). It is now abundantly clear that with normal cells TCGF can
only induce growth after the T-cells are activated. Only after anti-
gen/lectin activation are receptors for TCGF available. A schematic
illustration of these interactions is shown in Figure 1 and the properties of the normal cells in Table 1. For more detailed description
and references see the recent review [8].

**PROPOSED MECHANISM OF ACTION OF
T-LYMPHOCYTE GROWTH FACTOR**

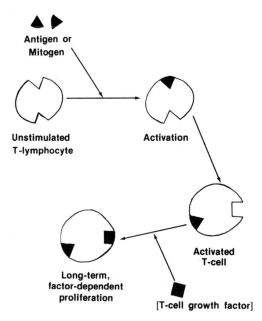

Figure 1. Simplified scheme for normal T-cell proliferation in response to antigen.

TABLE 1
Characteristics of Normal Cells Grown with TCGF for Long Periods

1. Source of cells	Normal blood or bone marrow
2. Morphology	Lymphoblast
3. Test for B-lymphoblast	Negative for immunoglobulins and for EBV
4. Histochemistry	Negative for myeloid (myeloperoxidase, chloroacetate esterase) and monocyte - macrophage (non-specific esterase) markers
5. Tests for T-cell markers	E-Rosette positive and functional mature T-cell assays (cytotoxic and helper T-cell activity) positive. Terminal transferase negative.
6. Initiation of growth	Requires PHA or antigen TCGF cannot initiate
7. Maintenance of growth	Requires TCGF
8. Karyotype	Remains normal diploid even after growth over one year

Nature of TCGF

Human TCGF was recently purified (4,5). The starting material was lymphocyte conditioned media obtained from cultured peripheral blood mononuclear cells which had been pooled from 1 unit of blood from multiple normal donors. The cells were cultured for a few days in the presence of PHA in serum free RPMI media. The media was filtered (Millipore), dialyzed, and macromolecules precipitated with $(NH_4)SO_4$ and this material formed the first fractions in the purification steps. Subsequent steps are summarized in Table 2 and published in detail elsewhere [4,5].

The known biochemical and biological properties of TCGF are summarized in Tables 3 and 4 respectively. An interesting feature of purified human TCGF is its lack of species specificity but apparent cell type specificity, interacting only with activated T-lymphocytes.

TABLE 2
Procedure for Purification of Human TCGF

---

1. Starting material: Ly-CM pooled from serum free media (RPMI-1640 with BSA) in which mononuclear cells had been treated with PHA. The media used was derived from incubations of 30 to 40 units of blood. This media is filtered through a millipire filter to remove membranous debris.

2. $(NH_4)_2 SO_4$ ppt (50-75% saturation) and dialysis

3. DEAE--sepharose column chromatography

4. Ultragel ACA--54 column chromatography

5. First preparative SDS--PAGE

6. Second preparative SDS--PAGE

TABLE 3
Biochemical Properties of Human TCGF

---

1. Sensitivity to treatments
    a. Boiling   +
    b. RNase   −
    c. DNase   −
    d. Trypsin   +
    e. Freezing[a]   −
    f. NEM   −
    g. DTT   −
    h. Hg Cl$_2$ −

2. Stabilized by
    a. PEG   +
    b. Albumin   +
    c. Glycerol   −

3. MW   12-13,000
                                  SDS-PAGE

4. PI   6.8

5. Tests for glycosyl moiety   −

---

[a]Stable with PEG

TABLE 4
Summary of Biological Properties of Human TCGF

1.	Origin	Released from a subset of mature T-cells but also requires macrophage in this process.
2.	Target cell	"Activated" T-cells (helper, suppresser, cytotoxic)
3.	Biological effect	Promotes growth of activated T-cells after binding to specific receptor.
4.	Species specificity	Very little. Human TCGF active on other primates, cows, cats, rodents.

Direct Growth of Neoplastic T-Cells with TCGF

Recently, we found that T cells from patients with leukemias and lymphomas of mature T-cells directly respond to TCGF [9]. This suggests that these cells differ from normal T-cells by maintaining TCGF receptors while normal cells must first be activated in vitro (unless, of course, there has been a recent substantial antigenic in vivo stimulation to the normal cells). This might mean that these neoplastic T-cells are chronically exposed to some antigens or that in the process of neoplastic transformation a membrane change occurs which makes available a previously "cryptic" TCGF receptor.

When crude TCGF was used growth of the neoplastic T-cells was generally maintained for only 3-6 weeks. There are inhibitors of TCGF activity in the crude and even partially purified fractions. These include interferon, PHA (which inhibits the long term growth effect of TCGF), and other unidentified substances. When the more purified TCGF was used growth was maintained, and in some cases cell lines independent of TCGF were established [9,10]. These cell lines were established from patients with cutaneous T-cell leukemias and lymphomas (Sezary syndrome and mycosis fungoides, respectively), and

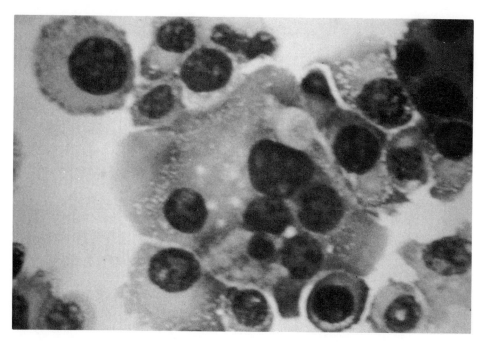

Figure 2. Light microscopy of Giemsa stained cultured Sezary leukemia T-cells. Note the giant multinucleated cell.

they have several interesting features. They have characteristics of mature T-cells (E-rosette positive) but also are positive for non-specific esterase, a macrophage marker. The cultured cells include 1-15% giant multinucleated cells often surrounded by smaller mono- or binucleated cells in rosette like fashion (Figure 2). Some cells have convoluted nuclei as Sezary lymphocytes. The chief characteristics are summarized in Table 5.

Some of the cultures which have been established as lines became constitutive producers of TCGF [11] which, of course, is the likely explanation for their becoming independent of exogenous TCGF. However, in some instances they also release other interesting molecules which effect growth of different kinds of cells and in different ways. For instance, activities such as colony stimulating activity for macrophage and granulocytes, interferon, and burst promoting activity for erythroid cell proliferation have been found released from one or more of these cell lines [11].

TABLE 5

Comparative Properties of Continuously Cultured Human T-Cells

Source of Cells	Requirements for Growth			Morphology	TdT[c]	EBV[d] IgG	E-Rosette	Acid Phosphatase	Non-specific Esterase	Chromosomes
	No Additions	TCGF Alone	TCGF and PHA Initiation							
Normal	-	-	+	Normal lymphoblasts	-	-	+	+ Mild granular cytoplasmic	-	Normal diploid
ALL[a]	- (rarely +)	+	+	Homogenous lymphoblasts- sometimes with multiple nucleoli in nucleus	-	-	+	++ Concentrated in Golgi region	-	Variable and like primary cells
CTCL[b]	- (rarely +)	+	+	Heterogenous giant multi-nucleated cells and other smaller lympho-blasts mono- or binucleated; some with con-voluted nuclei	-	-	+	+++ Diffuse intense reaction	Diffuse intense re-action in a few cells; majority-small para-nuclear cytoplasmic granule	Variable and like primary cells

[a]ALL means acute lymphoblastic leukemia--T-cell type.

[b]CTCL means cutaneous T-cell leukemia or lymphoma (Sezary or mycosis fungoides).

[c]TdT means terminal deoxyribonucleotidyl transferase.

[d]Tests for EBV were by assays for the EBV specific nuclear antigen.

Detection, Isolation, and Characterization
of a New Type-C Retrovirus (HTLV)

In the above discussion it was noted that some of the cultured T-cells
from patients with cutaneous T-cell leukemia or lymphoma became independent of TCGF apparently because they began to produce their own
TCGF. In some of these we noted releases of a type-C RNA tumor virus
[10,12-15]. The first isolate, called human T-cell leukemia (lymphoma)
virus strain CR (HTLV$_{CR}$), obtained from a patient with mycosis fungoides, has been studied most extensively and involved a collaboration
with Dr. John Minna and his colleagues Dr. A. Gazdar and Dr. P. Bunn
of the NCI-VA Clinical Oncology Branch. The cells were obtained from
an inguinal lymph node biopsy. Subsequently, independent clinical
specimens were obtained (blood samples) from which T-cells were grown
and HTLV$_{CR}$ again identified. At almost the same time we received a
blood sample from Dr. J. Rosenthal (Downstate Medical Center, New York)
obtained from a patient with Sezary leukemia. We established a cell
line and again identified a type-C virus termed HTLV$_{MB}$ (Figure 3).
Analyses of HTLV$_{CR}$ and HTLV$_{MB}$ revealed that they are highly related
to each other but distinct from previously isolated animal retroviruses [10,13-15].

We have distinguished the HTLV isolates from other viruses by 3
sets of tests: (1) The reverse transcriptase of HTLV was antigenic-
ally unrelated to reverse transcriptase of animal retroviruses by
enzyme neutralization tests [13,16]; (2) the P24 (major internal core
protein) of HTLV was distinguished from the major core proteins of
animal retroviruses by competition radioimmune assays [15]; (3) the
nucleotide sequences of HTLV were only distantly related to nucleotide
sequences of other viruses by liquid molecular hybridization [14].

Origin of HTLV and the Possible Role
of TCGF and HTLV in the Pathogenesis
of Lymphomas and Leukemias of Mature T-Cells

HTLV was chiefly found in cells which also release TCGF. It appears
from cell cloning studies carried out by Dr. M. Maeda in our laboratory that the leukemic cells which release TCGF also respond to it.

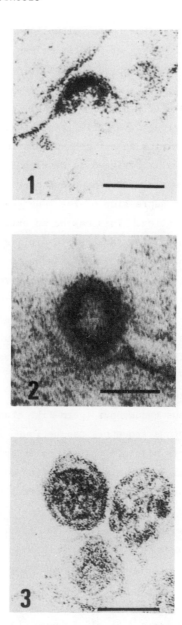

Figure 3. Electron micrograph of the type-C retrovirus, HTLV from CTCL-2 cells, the cell line described in Figure 2. Note the formation of a typical virus bud in panel 1 (top), the early formed virus in panel 2 (middle), and the mature released virions in panel 3 (bottom). The virus size is variable but approximates 1000 A°.

This seems different from the normal situation where most observations suggest to us that one subset of T-cells release TCGF while a separate set respond to it. This suggested the following model which my colleague Dr. F. Ruscetti and I have developed from these results (Figure 4). In this model an HTLV protein (presumably the envelope) interacts with a very specific group of T-cells (those which have receptors for the envelope). This mimics an antigen stimulation of blastogenesis. The T-cell is one normally designed to develop TCGF receptors and does so. However, promoter-like sequences contained in the integrated HTLV provirus triggers depression of the TCGF gene, leading to TCGF release and autostimulation. This may be an early step in the transformation. Subsequently, the increase in proliferation leads to an increased incidence of mutation with fixation of the transformed state. Virus expressing cells are selected against by immune mechanisms so that one may only rarely identify virus by the time overt leukemia occurs. Other initiators (non-viral) may be involved in the early stages of other forms of T-cell lymphomas and leukemias, but even in these cases abnormalities in TCGF production or response may be central to the pathogenesis of these diseases.

The natural "reservoir" of HTLV is unknown. We have shown that it is not an ubiquitous endogenous (germ-like transmitted) virus of man because no homologous sequences can be found in DNA from normal humans. However, it is possible that it is endogenous within select families, i.e., families with a predisposition for these diseases. This is testable. For instance, if it is germ-line transmitted we should find sequences in the DNA of normal cells from the mother or father of a patient with these diseases who himself has the virus. We should also find nucleotide sequences of HTLV in the DNA of normal cells of patients with the disease. Neither experiment has yet been done.

Recently, specific antibodies to HTLV were found in the sera of a few patients with cutaneous T-cell lymphoma [17]. One positive result was with serum from C. R., the first patient from whom HTLV was isolated. These antibodies were detected by both ELISA and RIP assays and in both cases competition assays showed remarkable speci-

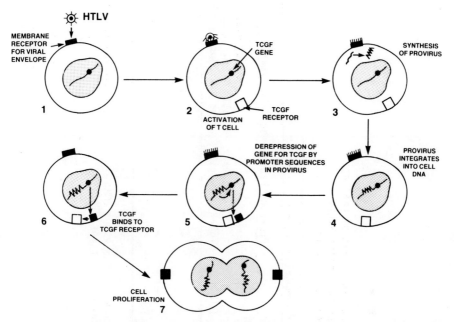

Figure 4. A schematic and simple model for the first stage of T-cell
leukemic transformation. We propose that the target cell is a mature
T-cell with an antigen receptor site, which in the case of a proposed
viral induced disease, recognizes an envelope protein of HTLV. This
leads to the recently known antigen effect of inducing the availability of receptors for TCGF. Concommitantly, nucleic acid sequences
contained in the HTLV genome which are integrated into the host cell
DNA include sequences which can act as promotors for expression of certain cell genes. (Much evidence suggests that this may be the case in
animal models with animal retroviruses.) We suggest that this leads
to an abnormal expression of the gene for TCGF. We think the available
data indicate that separate subsets of T-cells usually make and respond
to TCGF under normal circumstances. The above model of a cell both
making and responding to TCGF may lead to uncontrolled proliferation.
In turn, this may subsequently lead to an increase in the likelihood of
mutational events which "fix" the transformed state. Later in the progression of leukemogenesis cells which express virus may be selected
against by immune mechanisms, making and finding them rare and difficult
by the time of frank disease.

TABLE 7

Specificity of Natural Antibodies from Serum of Patients
with Cutaneous T-Cell Lymphoma Against HTLV:
Competition in RIP and ELISA Assays

| | Test of Competing Antigen | | | | | | | | | |
| | Proteins From Viruses | | | | | Proteins From Human Cell Lysates | | | | |
Patient Source of Serum Anti-body	FCS	BSA	HTLV$_{CR}$	HTLV$_{MB}$	Numerous Animal Retroviruses	HUT-102[a]	CTCL-2[a]	Normal T-Cells	Normal B-Cell Lines	Transformed T-Cell Lines Not Producing HTLV
CTCL-CR≠	−	−	+	+	−	+	+	−	−	−
CTCL-4≠	−	−	+	+	−	+	+	−	−	−

[a]Cell lines produce HTLV

CTCL-CR is the patient from whom cell line HUT-102 was established. The virus HTLV^{CR} was first isolated from these cells. CTCL-4 is another patient with a similar stage of disease as patient CTCL-CR.

ficity (see summary of specificity data in Table 6). The presence
of antibodies is perhaps more suggestive of an exogenous entry of
HTLV, i.e., by some kind of a poorly understood infection. However,
antibodies can occur to endogenous viruses so the question of its
origin must remain open. It will be important to look globally for
clusters of patients with these types of leukemias and lymphomas. A
careful study of disease clusters and of family studies combined with
information generated from molecular biological studies with HTLV
reagents may lead to a better understanding of the origin of these
diseases.

ACKNOWLEDGMENTS

Many of the studies here were carried out by colleagues in my laboratory. Notably, Dr. B. Poiesz, a former research associate postdoctoral in our laboratory made important contributions to the growth
of the neoplastic T-cells and to the early detection of HTLV. My
present coworker, Dr. F. Ruscetti, made significant contributions to
the biological work on TCGF and to growth of the T-cells and
Dr. J. Mier, formerly a research associate post-doctoral with us, to
the purification of TCGF. Several colleagues have contributed to the
analysis of HTLV, especially Dr. M. Reitz, Dr. H. Rho, and
Dr. V. Kalyanaraman. In addition, as mentioned in the text, a portion
of the work in the first virus isolate involving patient C. R. and
the cell line established from that patient, as well as all clinical
serum samples were in collaboration with Dr. J. Minna, Dr. P. Bunn,
and Dr. A. Gazdar of the NCI-VA Oncology Branch.

REFERENCES

1. Morgan, D. A., Ruscetti, F. W., and Gallo, R. C., *Science,*
    193:1007-1008 (1976).

2. Ruscetti, F. W., Morgan, D., and Gallo, R. C., *J. Immunol.,*
    119:131-138 (1977).

3. Smith, K., T-Cell Growth Factor: Present Status and Future
    Implications. In: Lymphokine Reports, Vol. II (E. Pick, ed.),
    Academic Press, in press.

4. Mier, J. W., and Gallo, R. C., *Proc. Nat. Acad. Sci., U.S.A.,*
    in press.

5. Mier, J. W., and Gallo, R. C., (submitted).

6. Riddick, D. H., and Gallo, R. C., *Cancer Res., 30:*2484-2492
    (1970).

7. Prival, J., Paran, M., Gallo, R. C., and Wu, A. M., *J. Natl.
    Cancer Inst., 53:*1583-1588 (1974).

8. Ruscetti, F. W., and Gallo, R. C., *Blood,* Editoral Review,
    *57:*379-394 (1981).

9. Poiesz, B. J., Ruscetti, F. W., Mier, J. W., Woods, A. M., and
    Gallo, R. C., *Proc. Nat. Acad. Sci., U.S.A.,* in press.

10. Gallo, R. C., Poiesz, B. J., and Ruscetti, F. W., Regulation of
    Human T-Cell Proliferation: T-Cell Growth Factor and Isolation
    of a New Class of Type-C Retroviruses from Human T-Cells. In:
    Modern Trends in Human Leukemia IV (R. Neth, K. Mannweiler,
    T. Graf, and R. C. Gallo, eds.), *Springer-Verlag Press,* in press.

11. Tarella, C., Ruscetti, F., Gazdar, A., Poiesz, B., and Gallo,
    R. C., submitted.

12. Poiesz, B. J., Ruscetti, F. W., Gazdar, A. F., Bunn, P. A.,
    Minna, J. D., and Gallo, R. C., *Proc. Nat. Acad. Sci., U.S.A.,*
    in press.

13. Poiesz, B. J., Ruscetti, F. W., Reitz, M. S., Kalyanaraman, V. S.,
    and Gallo, R. C., in preparation.

14. Reitz, M. S., Jr., Poiesz, B. J., Ruscetti, F. W., and Gallo,
    R. C., *Proc. Nat. Acad. Sci.,* U.S.A. *78:*1887-1891 (1981).

15. Kalyanaraman, V. S., Sarngadharan, M. G., Poiesz, B., Ruscetti,
    F. W., and Gallo, R. C., *J. Virology,*

16. Rho, H. M., Poiesz, B., Ruscetti, F. W., and Gallo, R. C.,
    Virology, in press.

17. Posner, L. E., Robert-Guroff, M., Kalyanaraman, V. S., Poiesz,
    B. J., Ruscetti, F. W., Bunn, P. A. Jr., and Gallo, R. C.,
    J. Experimental Med., in press.

PROPERTIES OF SARCOMA GROWTH FACTORS
PRODUCED BY SARCOMA VIRUS TRANSFORMED CELLS

Joseph E. De Larco
George J. Todaro

Laboratory of Viral Carcinogenesis
National Cancer Institute
Frederick Cancer Research Center
Frederick, Maryland

INTRODUCTION

Murine sarcoma virus (MSV) transformed cells have been characterized by a loss of measurable cell surface receptors for the growth stimulating polypeptide, epidermal growth factor, (EGF) [1,2]. The apparent loss of cell surface receptors occurs in both fibroblastic and epitheloid cells transformed by MSV [3]. The MSV-transformed cells release polypeptides into the medium that stimulate cell growth and initiate a phenotypic change in the morphology of untransformed monolayer cell cultures and also induce anchorage independent cell growth [2]. Several of these polypeptide, growth factors compete with EGF for its membrane receptors. These factors are specific for sarcoma virus-transformed cells in that neither supernatants from untransformed cells nor cells transformed by DNA tumor virus have detectable quantities of these EGF competing polypeptide growth factors. The major soft agar growth stimulating activity, sarcoma growth factor (SGF), has an apparent molecular weight of approximately 10,000 and will not stimulate the growth of cells lacking active EGF receptors.

Radiolabeled SGF is purified and characterized using human carcinoma cells that have a large number of EGF receptors. The EGF receptors are used as affinity sites for binding SGF. These studies show that the binding to and eluting from the EGF receptors yields a specific radiolabeled peptide as well as agar growth stimulating activity [4]. The specific binding to the EGF receptors rose from 0.1% of the input counts for the crude material to approximately 25% of the input counts for the twice cycled material. Cycling also provides a single iso-electric focusing band at pH 6.8 for the ^{125}I-SGF, whereas uncycled material had a heterogenous isoelectric profile. Cells lacking EGF receptors are unable to respond to the growth stimulating effects of this partially purified SGF [5]. It appears therefore, that SGF re-leased by MSV-transformed cells elicits its biologic effects via specific interaction with EGF membrane receptors.

To determine whether the SGF is a product of the sarcoma virus genome or a product of a cellular origin, the SGF-like peptide growth factor from a temperature sensitive Kirsten sarcoma virus transformed cell was investigated (ts-371 cl 5) [6]. At the temperature permis-sive for transformation (32°C) these cells display the transformed phenotype, lack measurable EGF receptors as determined by ^{125}I-EGF binding, grow in soft agar, and release SGF-like peptides; whereas at the nonpermissive temperature they display a flat morphology, have EGF receptors, and neither grow in soft agar nor release SGF-like peptides. The SGF-like growth factors released at the permissive temperature by cells transformed with this ts-sensitive mutant is compared with the cells transformed by the wild type sarcoma virus. Neither of these growth factors are temperature sensitive under the conditions of assay (65 C X 120 min.).

MATERIALS AND METHODS

Serum Free Conditioned Media

The cells were grown in roller bottles (Falcon #3027;850 cm^2) contain-ing Dulbecco's modification of Eagle's medium (DMEM) [7] with 10% calf serum (Colorado Serum Co.). The cells were washed once for 1 hour and again for 16 hours with 100 ml of serum-free Waymouth's medium

[8] (GIBCO, MD705/1). These washes were discarded and two subsequent serum-free 48-hour collections were harvested and are referred to as "conditioned media." The viability of the cells maintained either in a medium containing 10% serum or in serum-free for 5 days with 4 changes of medium was greater than 80%, as determined by trypan blue exclusion. The "sarcoma-conditioned media" were clarified by centrifugation at 100,000 X g for 45 minutes. The supernate was concentrated 20-fold in a hollow fiber apparatus (Amicon;DC2), and dialyzed against 5 changes consisting of 5 volumes each of 1% acetic acid. This material was lyophilized and extracted with 1 M acetic acid. One percent of the volume of the starting conditioned media was used. The extract was clarified by centrifugation at 100,000 X g for 30 minutes. Approximately 90% of this 1 M acetic acid extract was chromatographed through a Bio-Gel P-60 column (5 X 90 cm) that had been equilibrated in and eluted with 1 M acetic acid. The column was run at 4° C at a flow rate of 15 ml/hr and 15 ml fractions were collected unless otherwise stated. Aliquots were lyophilized for protein determinations [9], EGF competition, stimulation of thymidine incorporation, and soft agar growth activity.

The EGF was isolated from male mouse salivary glands [10]. This peptide was labeled with ^{125}I using a modification of the original chloramine-T method [11]. Between 10 and 20 ug of lyophilized protein were dissolved in 50 ul of 0.4 M sodium phosphate, pH 7.5, and 2 mCi of ^{125}I, as the sodium salt, were added. The reactions were initiated by adding 5 ul of chloramine-T solution (100 ug/ml); 2 minutes later an additional 5 ul aliquot was added, and after an additional 1.5 minutes the third and last 5 ul aliquot of chloramine-T was added. One minute after the last addition of chloramine-T, the iodinations were stopped by adding 100 ul of saturated tyrosine in 0.01 M Tris-HCl, pH 8.4. The iodinated proteins were separated from the reagents by passing the mixtures over columns (0.7 X 14 cm) of Sephadex G-15 equilibrated in an eluted with phosphate buffered saline (PBS). Bovine serum albumin (Pentex-Cystallized) (BSA) was added to the peak tubes to give a final concentration of 5 mg/ml, the fractions were pooled, and small aliquots were stored frozen at -20°C.

Assays for EGF Bindings and for Radioreceptor Competitions

The ^{125}I-EGF binding assays were performed on subconfluent cell cultures of Mv-1-Lu (CCL64, American Type Culture Collection). Cells were seeded at 2.5 X 10^4 cells per 16 mm well (Linbro Cat. No. 76-033-05) in DMEM containing 10% calf serum. After 24 hours the medium was removed and the cells were washed twice with binding buffer (DMEM containing 1 mg/ml BSA and 50 mM N,N-bis-(2-hydroxyethyl)-2-aminoethane-sulfonic acid (BES), ajusted to pH 6.8). [12]. ^{125}I-EGF bindings were initiated by adding 200 u liters of ^{125}I-EGF solution (2 ng/ml). The bindings were continued for 1 hour at room temperature. The unbound radiolabeled EGF was removed and the monolayers were washed three times with binding buffer to remove traces of unbound labeled EGF. The radiolabeled ligand bound was quantitated by lysing the cells (0.01 M Tris.HCl, pH 7.4 containing 0.5% sodium dodecyl sulfate and 0.005 M EDTA) and counting the lysate in a gamma counter. Nonspecific binding was estimated by determining the amount of cell-bound radioactivity in the presence of a large excess of unlabeled EGF (10 ug/ml). The specific binding is obtained by subtracting the nonspecific binding from the total binding.

Assay for Growth-Promoting Activity

Serum-deprived, subconfluent normal rat kidney cells were prepared for this assay by trypsinizing the fibroblastic clone 49F [3]. They were seeded at 2.5 X 10^4 cells per 16 mm well (Linbro Cat. No. 76-033-05) in DMEM containing 10% calf serum. After 24 hours the medium was removed; the cells were washed with fresh serum-free medium and then incubated with 1 ml per well of Waymouth's medium containing 0.1% calf serum. Three days later, 0.1 ml of binding buffer containing the sample to be tested was added. Sixteen hours after the addition, the cells were exposed for 8 hours to 2.5 uCi of ^{3}H-thymidine (NEN; NET-027, 6.7 ci/mM). The medium containing the radiolabeled thymidine was removed, and the cultures were washed twice with 1 ml of DMEM containing 100 ug/ml unlabeled thymidine and incubated for 30 min.

After the incubation, the monolayers were washed three times, the
cells were disrupted with lysing buffer, and the DNA was precipitated
by adding the lysate to 3 vol. of cold 10% trichloroacetic acid. The
precipitated DNA was removed by filtration (Millipore; HA, 0.45 uM);
the filters were dried and added to counting vials with 5 ml of
toluene/Liquifluor (NEN, NEF 903), and the radioactivity measured in
a liquid scintillation counter (Beckman, LS-250).

Soft Agar Growth Assay

Soft agar assays were performed using the NRK fibroblastic clone 49F.
Agar plates were prepared in 60-mm tissue culture dishes (Falcon,
3003) by first applying a 2 ml base layer of 0.5% agar (Difco, Agar
Noble) in DMEM containing 10% calf serum. Over this basal layer, an
additional 2 ml layer of 0.3% agar was added to the above medium containing the appropriate concentration of protein, and 1×10^4 indicator cells. These dishes were incubated at $37°C$ in a humidified atmosphere of 5% CO_2 in air. Colonies were measured unfixed and unstained
using an inverted microscope. Colonies with greater than 50 cells
were scored as positive unless otherwise stated.

Receptor Affinity Purification of EGF-like Molecules

The human carcinoma line, A431, which is known to have a large number
of EGF receptors, was used in order to preferentially bind EGF-like
molecules from an iodinated stock containing SGF. The A431 cells
were fixed to tissue culture dishes by treating them with a 5% solution
of formaldehyde in PBS for 5 minutes. The formaldehyde solution was
removed from the cells, which were then washed four times with PBS,
and twice with binding buffer. The Bio-Gel P-60 pool II was radioiodinated to a specific activity of 73 mCi/ug. The iodinated material
was diluted in binding buffer and bound to fixed A431 cells for 90
minutes at 22°C. The unbound material was removed and saved for further binding. The cells were washed four times with binding buffer
and the bound material was eluted from the cells using three 1 ml

washes of 0.1% acetic acid. The acetic acid was lyophilized. The
bound and eluted material (s) were reconstituted in binding buffer.
The three fractions, (1) untreated, (2) unbound, and (3) bound and
eluted, were tested for their ability to bind to A431 cells using the
standard binding conditions.

Heat Treatment

Lyophilized pools of the materials to be tested for temperature sensitivity were dissolved and diluted in binding buffer that had been
neutralized with 0.5 $\underline{M}$ trisodium phosphate. Two aliquots of one ml
were taken from each sample and placed in a plastic capped tube (Falcon
#2063). One tube of each, the control, was kept on ice while the
other aliquot of each was heated in a 65°C water bath for 2 hours.
After heating, these tubes were placed in an ice bath. The bioassays
were run on all samples simultaneously.

RESULTS

The human carcinoma cell line, A431, has an exceptionally large number
of epidermal growth factor (EGF) receptors [13]. A Scatchard plot
for EGF binding to A431 cells generates a linear plot, and at saturating EGF concentrations these cells bind approximately 2.2×10^6 molecules of EGF per cell. In contrast, Scatchard plots obtained using
a fibroblastic normal rat kidney (NRK) clone show they only bind approximately 2.4×10^4 molecules of EGF per cell at saturating concentrations of EGF [4]. Taking advantage of these findings and those
previously described which show that SGF acts through the EGF receptor
[5], we decided to test whether SGF could be purified using formalin-
fixed A431 human carcinoma cells to selectively enrich for this growth
factor. The starting material or crude SGF used in this purification
was the 10,000 molecular weight peptide pool obtained from a Bio-Gel
P-60 chromatography [2].

      The A431 cells were fixed with formaldehyde in tissue culture
dishes and then used to specifically bind either mouse salivary gland

EGF or SGF produced by MSV-transformed cells. The unbound material
from these preparations was removed, the cells washed several times,
and the bound growth factors dissociated from their receptors with
dilute acid. The materials released retain their biological activities
and can rebind to their receptors.

Table 1 shows the ability of different radiolabeled SGF preparations to bind to and be eluted from A431 cells. After two cycles of
binding and eluting, the remaining counts bound with a much higher
efficiency to A431 cells. In the case of the twice-cycled material,
approximately 24% of the input counts bound specifically to the A431
cells; whereas only 0.12% of the input counts from the crude SGF bound
specifically to the A431 cells. The ratio of specific to nonspecific
binding for SGF also increased with cycling from 0.18 for the uncycled
material to 18.7 in the case of the twice cycled material. The re-
cycled radiolabeled-SGF did not bind to a clone of mouse 3T3 cells
which lack EGF receptors [14] (data not shown).

TABLE 1

Purification of ^{125}I-SGF Using Binding and Elution
from an EGF Receptor-Rich Cell

Material	$\dfrac{\text{Specific Binding}}{\text{Nonspecific Binding}}$	Percent of input dpm Bound
Bio-Gel P-60 pool II	0.18	0.12
After the first cycle	5.6	2.8
After the second cycle	18.7	23.9

When 12 ug of unlabeled crude SGF was cycled over fixed A431
cells in a 100 mm tissue culture dish as described in Materials and
Methods, the receptors were able to bind and release the biological
activity. Table 2 shows that the portion which was bound to and eluted
from the fixed cells contained over 90% of the activity found in the
untreated SGF preparation. If one assumes the percentage of unlabeled
peptides which bound to the fixed A431 cells is similar to that for
the radiolabeled peptides (Table 1), then there was considerably less

TABLE 2
Soft Agar Growth Stimulation
By Cycled Bio-Gel P-60 Pool II SGF Preparations

Preparation	Percent of Seeded Cells Forming Colonies With Greater Than 50 Cells
Untreated Pool II at a final concentration of 1.2 ug/ml	60
Pool II unbound to fixed A431 cells	4
Pool II bound to and eluted from fixed A431 cells	55
Binding buffer unbound to fixed A431 cells	0
Binding buffer bound to and eluted from fixed A431 cells	0

Ten milliliters of either binding buffer of binding buffer containing 12 ug/ml of Pool II SGF was bound to fixed A431 cells for 45 min at room temperature. The unbound material was then transferred to another dish of fixed A431 cells and bound for an additional 45 min. The plates were each washed twice with serum-free Waymouth's medium and PBS before eluting the "bound materials" from the fixed cells. The eluted materials were lyophilized and redissolved in a volume of binding buffer equal to that of the unbound material. Soft agar assays were set up using the above materials at a 1:10 dilution and read after 13 days.

than 5 ng per ml of peptide from SGF pool II in the soft agar assay of the bound and eluted material. In the controls, which consisted of binding buffer cycled over fixed A431 cells, neither the "unbound" nor the "bound" materials had any soft agar growth stimulating activity.

To contrast the differences in homogeneity of the radiolabeled peptide preparations prior to and after cycling over fixed A431 cells, isoelectric-focusing was performed. In Figure 1 we show isoelectric focusing columns run on ^{125}I-labeled EGF and iodinated preparations of crude SGF before and after cycling on fixed A431 cell monolayers. Isoelectric focusing of the ^{125}I-labeled EGF preparation prior to

purification using fixed A431 cells (Figure 1A) gave two sharp peaks.
The smaller peak has a pI of 3.8 and the larger peak has a pI of 4.4.
The labeled EGF that had been bound to and eluted from fixed cells
gave a single sharp peak upon isoelectric focusing which had a pI of
4.4 (Figure 1B); this value is consistent with that previously published for EGF [15]. In contrast, isoelectric focusing of iodinated
crude SGF gave a heterodisperse profile with the majority of the
labeled material having acidic pI's (Figure 1C). The radiolabeled
peptide(s) from crude SGF which was bound to and eluted from the
fixed A431 cells, however, gave a sharp peak upon isoelectric focusing
which had a pI of between 6.8 and 7.0 (Figure 1D).

To test if isoelectric focusing could be used preparatively to
purify the growth stimulating activity, an experiment was performed
in which unlabeled crude SGF was isoelectric focused with carrier
^{125}I-SGF that had been purified by cycling on EGF receptor-rich human
carcinoma cells (Figure 2). The fractions were tested for their
ability to stimulate both the colony formation in soft agar and cell
division as measured by the incorporation of ^{3}H-thymidine into the
DNA of growth arrested fibroblastic NRK cell monolayers. These major
growth activities comigrated with the radioactivity from the cycled
^{125}I-SGF and is found in a narrow region with a pI of between 6.8 and
7.0. Isoelectric focusing, then, can be used to further purify the
growth factor from crude preparations with the retention of biological
activity.

The SGF obtained by two cycles of binding to and eluting from
A431 receptors was compared with the original crude material and with
EGF on 10-30% polyacrylamide gradient gels. The results are shown
in Figure 3. Mouse viral p30 in slots A and H (molecular weight approximately 30,000) and porcine relaxin in slots B and G (molecular
weight approximately 6,000) were used as ^{125}I-labeled marker proteins.
It is seen that the purified SGF runs as though it is slightly heavier
than the relaxin standard. The EGF preparation migrated slower than
the relaxin standard. There was no detectable difference in the migration patterns of the untreated EGF, slot C, and the EGF that had
been bound to and eluted from fixed A431 cells, slot D. There was,

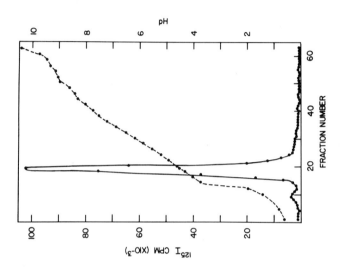

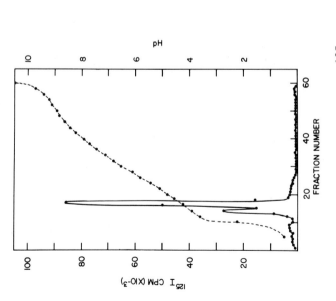

Figure 1. Isoelectric focusing of 125I-labeled peptides. Isoelectric focusing was performed using a 110 ml LKB column. A 1% solution of H_2SO_4 in 60% sucrose (w/v) was layered at the anode followed by a 40% to 0% (w/v) sucrose gradient containing 1% LKB ampholine ampholytes, pH3.5-10. The lyophilized 125I-labeled sample was resuspended in 1 ml of water mixed with 1 ml of the dense portion of the gradient and applied near the middle of the column. A 1% solution of NaOH was layered on top of the gradient in contact with the cathode. The column was run at 300 volts for 48 h at 4°C after which time 2 ml fractions were collected from the bottom of the column and the pH and content of 125I-labeled material of each fraction was measured.

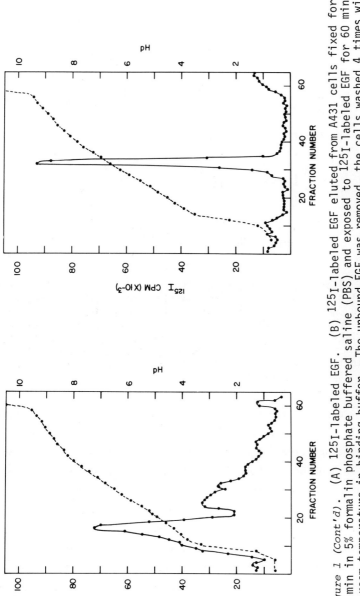

Figure 1 (Cont'd). (A) 125I-labeled EGF. (B) 125I-labeled EGF eluted from A431 cells fixed for 10 min in 5% formalin phosphate buffered saline (PBS) and exposed to 125I-labeled EGF for 60 min at room temperature in binding buffer. The unbound EGF was removed, the cells washed 4 times with binding buffer, and the bound material eluted with three washes of 0.1% acetic acid in water. (C) 125I-labeled crude SGF. (D) 125I-labeled SGF eluted from formalin-fixed A431 cells described in (B).

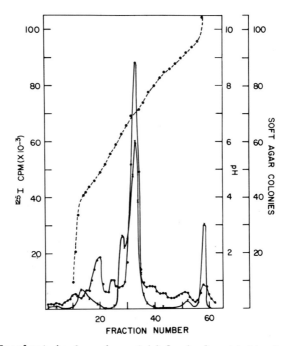

Figure 2. Isoelectric focusing of biological activity from crude SGF.
125I-labeled SGF eluted from formalin-fixed A431 cells, as described
in Fig. 1B, was applied to an isoelectric focusing column with 100 ugm
crude SGF from the 10,000 molecular weight region of a Bio-Gel P-60
column. Isoelectric focusing was performed as described in the legend
to Figure 1. A 100 ul aliquot of each indicated column fraction was
diluted in 1 M acetic acid, lyophilized and tested for soft agar
growth as described previously.

however, a marked difference between the migration pattern of the uncycled SGF, slot E, and SGF that had been cycled on fixed A431 cells,
slot F. The uncycled SGF migrated as a broad diffuse band that appeared as a doublet on the original X-ray film, whereas the cycled
SGF migrated as a sharp band centered with the diffuse band seen in
the uncycled pool II material. Both purified EGF and EGF cycled on
A431 cells ran as slightly heavier than SGF. This result is in contrast to their behavior on the Sephadex G-50 gel filtration system,
where SGF appears to be heavier than EGF. Using Bio-Gel P-60 chromatography (a polyacrylamide gel), SGF elutes as a peptide with an apparent molecular weight of approximately 10,000, while EGF adsorbs to

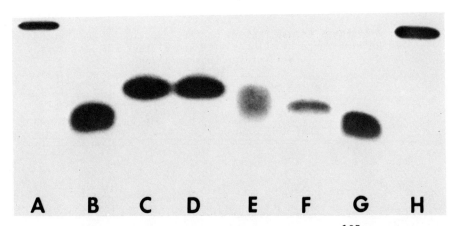

Figure 3. SDS-polyacrylamide gel electrophoresis of ^{125}I-labeled EGF and SGF before and after purification by cycling on formalin-fixed A431 cells. ^{125}I-labeled peptides: (A) Rauscher murine leukemia virus major structural protein, p30; (B) porcine relaxin; (C) EGF; (D) EGF bound to and eluted from A431 cells; (E) crude SGF; (F) SGF bound to and eluted from formalin fixed A431 cells; (G) porcine relaxin; and (H) Rauscher p30. Samples were heated for 2 min at 90°C in sample buffer (0.0625 M Tris-hydrochloride, pH 6.7, 1% SDS, 10% glycerol and 1% bromopherol blue) and electrophoresed through a 10-30% SDS-polyacrylamide gradient gel in a Tris-glycine-SDS buffer system [16]. Radioactive peptides were visualized by autoradiography using Kodak NS-5T film. ^{125}I-labeled Rauscher p30 (30,000) (A and H) and porcine relaxin (6,000) (B and G) were included as molecular weight markers.

the column and is eluted after the salt peak [10]. In each of these systems, however, it is clear that the active component of SGF is not mouse salivary gland EGF, but is a recognizably different peptide.

   To test whether EGF receptors are required for the biologic activity of SGF, clones derived from 3T3 cells that lack EGF receptors were tested. These clones were generously provided by Dr. Harvey Herschman (UCLA). They had been selected by stimulating the highly passaged 3T3 culture in the presence of colchicine [14]. While 3T3 itself are responsive to the mitogenic action of EGF, the selected clone, NR6/6, was neither responsive to the mitogenic action of EGF nor did it have detectable EGF receptors [15]. 3T3 cells and the NR6/6 clone were tested in parallel for their response to calf serum and to a number of purified growth factors, including mouse EGF [10, 16] and SGF. The parental clone, 3T3/8, responded to all of the growth

TABLE 3
Effect of Various Growth Factors on the Induction of DNA Synthesis
in Resting Mouse 3T3 Clones with and without EGF Receptors
^{3}H-Thymidine Incorporation
$(X\ 10^{-3})$

Test Cells Additions	3T3/8 (EGF-R$^+$)	NR6/6 (EGF-R$^-$)	% of Control Ratio of H^3-Thymidine Incorporation EGF-R$^+$ cells[a]
None	2.4	2.8	---
EGF(10 ng/ml)	33.5	3.1	<1
SGF(1 ug/ml)	63.7	2.9	<1
Calf serum (600 ug/ml)	55.3	63.7	115
FGF(10 ng/ml)	31.5	47.3	153
MSA(10 ng/ml)	18.2	14.3	73
H-MSA (200 ng/ml)	23.5	16.2	64

[a]The percent of the control thymidine incorporation was calculated
by multiplying the amount of ^{3}H-thymidine incorporated into stimulated NR6/6 cells above the background cells (cells to which no a
additions were made) by 100 and dividing this product by the amount
of ^{3}H-thymidine incorporated into the stimulated 3T3/8 cells above
that found in unstimulated background cells. % of control

^{3}H-thy. incorp.=

$$\frac{(^3\text{H-thy. incorp. by NR6/6 stim.} - {^3}\text{H-thy. incorp. by NR6/6 cont.}) \times 100}{(^3\text{H-thy. incorp. by 3T3/8 stim.} - {^3}\text{H-thy. incorp. by 3T3/8 cont.})}$$

factors tested, as determined by ^{3}H-thymidine incorporation into DNA
(Table 3). The NR6/6 clone, on the other hand, responded to all of
the growth factors except EGF and SGF. DNA synthesis was stimulated
in both clones when they were treated with calf serum [16], fibroblast
growth factor (EGF) [17], multiplication stimulating activity (MSA)
derived from rat liver cells [18,19], or the MSA-like activity released
from a human fibrosarcoma line [20]. The cells were also tested for
their ability to grow in soft agar in the presence of SGF. In the

soft agar assay, the 3T3/8 cells responded readily by developing a
high percentage of large colonies (>50%) when treated with SGF whereas
the EGF receptor negative cell, NR6/6, did not respond at all. The
above results suggest EGF receptors are required for SGF to exert
its biologic effect in mouse 3T3 cells.

Table 4 shows that the sarcoma virus-transformed cells, transformed by the Kirsten sarcoma virus mutant, Ts371 clone 5, show rapid
alterations in their available cell surface receptors when shifted
from permissive to nonpermissive temperatures. The cells were grown
for several days at a permissive temperature, 36°C, and then sifted
for a 24 hour period to 32°C, 36°C and 39°C, the latter being nonpermissive for expression of the transformed phenotype [6]. After 24

TABLE 4
Effect of Temperature at which Cells have Grown
on ^{125}I-EGF Binding

	Previous Day At	EGF Bound
TS371 c15	32°	1,470
	36°	3,940
	39°	10,970
Untransformed NRK	32°	8,700
	36°	9,500
	39°	8,300
KiSV transformed NRK	32°	350
	36°	200
	39°	260

hours, the cells were assayed for EGF receptors, as previously described. Whereas the cells transformed by wild type virus show essentially no receptors at any of the temperatures, the cells transformed
by the mutant viruses show a greatly increased number of receptors
at 39°C, comparable, in fact, to those found on the untransformed
parental cells. At 32°C, however, they show only 10 to 20% the number
of receptors shown at 39°C, and cells maintained at 36°C have repeat-

edly expressed an intermediate number of available EGF receptors.
The conclusion from these experiments are that the transformed cells
have the capability of producing EGF cell surface receptors. The
shift to the nonpermissive temperature, then, would involve the rapid
inactivation or disappearance of a product, presumably a protein, that
blocks EGF receptor availability.

Table 5 shows that the temperature-sensitive mutant-transformed
cells are able to respond to SGF at the nonpermissive temperature.
In soft agar assays they are comparable to their untransformed parental
cells in their ability to respond to SGF. This experiment shows that
the defect at the nonpermissive temperature is not the lack of ability
to respond to SGF.

TABLE 5
Growth Stimulation by SGF of Normal and TS Mutants
Transformed Cells at the Non-permissive Temperature

	Temp.	Agar Colony Formation
TS371 c15	32°	>500
	36°	>500
	39°	5
+ SGF (20 ug/ul)	39°	150
NRK	32°	0
	36°	0
	39°	0
+ SGF (20 ug/ml)	39°	70
KiSV transformed NRK	32°	>500
	36°	>500
	39°	>500

To determine whether SGF-like growth factors released by MSV-
transformed cells are a product of the sarcoma virus genome or the
host cell genome, the SGF-like peptides from a wild type Kirsten sarcoma virus transformed NRK cell (KNRK) was compared with that from a

temperature sensitive Kirsten sarcoma virus transformed NRK cell (ts-371 cl 5). Serum free conditioned media were collected from these sarcoma virus transformed clones, and their acid soluble peptides were separated over an acidic Bio-Gel P-60 column [2]. The results of the column runs are illustrated in Figure 4. The results of the chromatography on the acid soluble material from the serum free Waymouth's media conditioned by the KNRK is illustrated in Figure 4A. The protein concentration is shown as the solid line connecting the filled circles. The stimulation of ^{3}H-thymidine incorporation is seen as the solid line connecting the open circles; the soft agar colony forming activity is illustrated by the broken line connecting the x's. There are several peaks of biological activities; however, the major peak of agar growth stimulating activity eluted in fraction 69 and has an approximately apparent molecular weight of 10,000. In this case approximately 60% of the test cells formed colonies of 50 cells or greater. The ratio of thymidine stimulating activity to agar growth is the reverse of that found in the other peaks. The final concentration of protein added from the column fractions in this peak is approximately 1.5 micrograms per ml.

The serum free conditioned media was collected from the temperature sensitive clone that had been maintained at the permissive temperature (32°C). Since the specific activity of the conditioned media from this clone was less than that of the wild type transformant, a higher concentration of protein was used in these assays, and colonies greater than 8 cells rather than 50 were scored as positives. The major peak of soft agar growth stimulating activity was eluted in fraction 71 and corresponds to an apparent molecular weight of approximately 10,000. This is similar to the Moloney sarcoma virus transformed murine cell [2] and the Kirsten transformed NRK cell. The protein concentrations used in the assays performed on the peak tubes contain approximately 10 micrograms per ml.

To determine if the major growth activity present in the media conditioned by NRK cells transformed with a temperature-sensitive sarcoma virus (ts-371 cl 5) is itself temperature sensitive, and therefore potentially responsible for the ts-properties of this transformed cell,

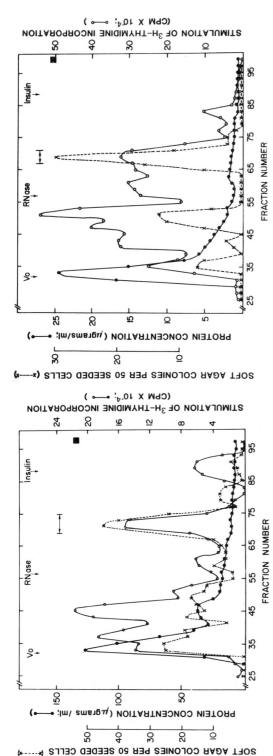

Figure 4. Bio-Gel P-60 chromatography of serum free conditioned media. The monolayers of cells were washed twice with serum free Weymouth's Media (8), once for an hour and the second time for 16 hours, and these were discarded. An additional two 48-hour harvests of serum free mediawere collected, clarified, concentrated, lyophilized, and extracted with 1 M acetic acid. The extracts were chromatographed using columns of Bio-Gel P-60 develpoed in 1 M acetic acid. Aliquots were lyophilized from the odd numbered fractions for protein determination. Second aliquots were taken from the same fractions, lyophized under sterile conditions, and dissolved in sterile binding buffer for use in the biological assays: 3H-thymidine incorporations (0-0), soft-agar growthassays (x—x) and EGF competitions (data not shown). The concentration of protein used in the bicassays is graphed (●-●). The assays were performed in duplicate and the values graphed represent the averages minus the appropriate blank. For the 3H-thymidine incorporation studies, the unstimulated cells served as the blank (binding buffer control), and cells stimulated by adding calf serum to a final concentration of 2% served as a reference (seen on the right of each figure as a solid square). The controls for EGF competition were 125I-EGF (2 ng/ml) plus unlabeled EGF (10 ug/ml) for the blank, to correct for nonspecific binding and background. 125I-EGF (2 ng/ml) and binding buffer for the positive and machine background. The soft-agar assays were scored 10 days after seeding.

A.) KNRK

B.) ts-371 cl 5

the activity present between the double headed arrow in Figure 4B was
pooled and tested along with the equivalent pool of activity present
in the media conditioned by NRK cell transformed by a wild type Kirsten
sarcoma virus (KNRK) (Fig. 4A). The results of these experiments are
found in Table 6. In comparing ts-371 cl 5 heated and unheated ali-

TABLE 6
Effects of Heating on the Biological Activity of Growth Factors
Released by Cells Transformed by Either a Wild Type KiSV
or a Temperature Sensitive (ts-371) KiSV

Source of Growth Factor	Stimulation of ^{3}H-Thymidine Incorporation cpm Above Control		Percent of 49F Cells That Formed Soft Agar Colonies[a]	
ts-371	dilution		dilution	
	1:4	30,651	1:1	75
	1:16	4,758	1:4	62
ts-371 heated[b]	1:4	28,588	1:1	76
	1:16	6,119	1:4	61
KNRK	1:3	135,721	1:3	70
	1:15	28,892	1:15	52
			1:75	4
KNRK heated[b]	1:3	129,766	1:3	66
	1:15	26,552	1:15	40
			1:75	8

[a]Colonies were scored 10 days after seeding. Those colonies
larger than approximately 20 cells were scored as positive.
[b]Heat treatment was carried out for 120 min in a water bath
maintained at 65°C. The samples were adjusted to pH 7.0 before
heating.

quots for their ability to stimulate thymidine incorporation, it appears there are little if any differences at either dilution. The
soft agar growth stimulating activity was also insensitive to this
heat treatment step as performed (samples were heated in a 65°C water
bath for 120 min at pH 7.0). The results from the heat treatment of

the equivalent factor(s) obtained from KNRK were quite similar, indicating the "SGF" obtained from the cell transformed by the temperature sensitive sarcoma virus is no more "temperature sensitive", under the conditions tested, than that obtained from the cell transformed by the wild type sarcoma virus.

DISCUSSION

A model consistent with these observations is the production and release by MSV-transformed cells of an EGF-like peptide factor or factors which are able to bind to and block cellular EGF receptors, and act as mitogens either on the cells producing them or on other cells having functional receptors capable of binding these factors. This could account for both the lack of measurable EGF receptors on the MSV-transformed cells as well as for the lowered serum requirement for MSV-transformed cells.

The data presented in this communication are consistent with the above model in that MSV-transformed cells produce at least one EGF-like peptide (SGF) which is capable of binding to and blocking EGF receptors. Using the EGF receptor to purify this peptide(s), the biological activity copurifies with the EGF receptor-binding activity. This factor from MSV-transformed cells has both similarities and differences when its properties are compared to mouse submaxillary gland EGF. It binds to EGF receptors with an affinity similar to EGF, and they both stimulate cell division in serum-depleted cells. They differ in that EGF has a more acidic pI (4.4) than SGF (6.8), they migrate differently in both SDS polyacrylamide gel electrophoresis and acetic acid (gel permeation) chromatography, and EGF will not stimulate anchorage independent growth while SGF will.

The above results demonstrate that SGF can be purified by taking advantage of its ability to reversibly interact with EGF membrane receptors on fixed cells. The purified peptide(s) has EGF receptor-competing activity as well as growth stimulating activity. The fixed human carcinoma cells, then, could be used to purify yet unknown growth factors that interact with the EGF receptor system.

The temperature sensitive MSV virus-transformed cells maintained at the permissive temperature of 32°C exhibit the transformed phenotype and either lack or have a greatly decreased number of available EGF receptors. If the media is changed and the cells are then incubated at the nonpermissive temperature (39°C), they begin to flatten out and their available EGF receptors begin to reappear within a day. The release of SGF-like growth factors by these transformed cells is also temperature dependent. The cells maintained at the permissive temperature release the SGF-like peptides whereas those maintained at the nonpermissive temperature do not. An obvious question arising from these studies is the origin of the growth factors released by sarcoma virus transformed cells. Are they direct viral products or are they host cell gene products that are controlled by the product of the sarcoma gene? If the growth factors which are able to confer the transformed phenotype on untransformed cells are viral gene products, one might expect them to be temperature sensitive when obtained from cells that are transformed by a sarcoma virus which is temperature sensitive with respect to transformation. If they are products of the host cell, they would be no more temperature sensitive than the growth factors isolated from cells transformed by the wild type virus. The regulation of their expression would, however, be temperature dependent and at the nonpermissive temperature the ts-sarcoma gene product would be inactivated and therefore unable to stimulate the host's expression of these growth factors. Recently, several groups have shown the src products from both avian and mammalian sarcoma virus exhibits an unusual protein kinase activity and, when kinase activities of temperature sensitive viruses were examined, they were shown to be more readily heat inactivated than the kinases of the wild type viruses [21,22, 23, and 24]. The SGF-like factor released by the ts-sarcoma virus transformed cells is extremely heat stable compared to the kinases and is no more temperature sensitive, under the conditions assayed, than the SGF-like factor released by cells transformed by the wild type sarcoma virus. This data suggests the SGF-like peptides produced and released by sarcoma virus transformed cells are not direct products of the murine sarcoma genomes, but rather the expression of cellular genes that are normally suppressed.

REFERENCES

1. Todaro, G. J., De Larco, J. E., and Cohen, S., Transformation
    by murine and feline sarcoma viruses specifically blocks binding
    of epidermal growth factor to cells, *Nature 264:*26-31 (1976).

2. De Larco, J. E. and Todaro, G. J., Growth factors from murine
    sarcoma virus-transformed cells, *Proc. Nat. Acad. Sci., U.S.A.,*
    *75:*4001-4005 (1978).

3. De Larco, J. E. and Todaro, G. J., Epithelioid and fibroblastic
    rat kidney cell clones: Epidermal growth factor (EGF) receptors
    and the effect of mouse sarcoma virus transformation, *J. Cell.*
    *Physiol. 94:*335-342 (1978).

4. De Larco, J.E., Reynolds, R., Carlberg, K., Engle, C. and Todaro,
    G., Sarcoma growth factor from mouse sarcoma virus-transformed
    cells. Purification by binding and elution from epidermal growth
    factor receptor-rich cells, *J. Biol. Chem. 255:*3685-3690 (1980).

5. De Larco, J. E. and Todaro, G. J., Sarcoma growth factor (SGF):
    specific binding to epidermal growth factor (EGF) membrane recep-
    tors, *J. Cell. Physiol. 102:*267-277 (1980).

6. Shih, T. Y., Weeks, M. O., Young, H. A. and Scolnick, E. M.,
    P-21 of Kirsten murine sarcoma virus is thermolabile in a viral
    mutant temperature sensitive for the maintenance of transforma-
    tion, *J. Virol. 31:*546-556 (1979).

7. Dulbecco, R., and Freeman, G., Plaque production by the polyoma
    virus, *Virology 8:*396-397 (1959).

8. Kitos, P. A., Sinclair, R., and Waymouth, C., Glutamine metabolism
    by animal cells growing in a synthetic medium, *Exp. Cell Res.*
    *27:*335-342 (1962).

9. Lowry, O. H., Rosebrough, N. J., Farr, A. L. and Randall, R. J.,
    Protein measurements with the folin phenol reagent, *J. Biol.*
    *Chem. 193:*265-275 (1951).

10. Savage, C. R., and Cohen, S., Epidermal growth factor and a new
    derivative. Rapid isolation procedures and biological and chemi-
    cal characterization, *J. Biol. Chem. 247:*7609-7611 (1972).

11. Greenwood, F. C., Hunter, W. M. and Glover, J. S., The prepara-
    tion of ^{131}I-labeled human growth hormone of high specific radio-
    activity, *Biochem. J. 8* :114-123 (1963).

12. De Larco, J. E. and Todaro, G. J., Membrane receptors for murine
    leukemia viruses: Characterization using the purified viral enve-
    lope glycoprotein, gp71, *Cell 8:*365-371 (1976).

13. Fabricant, R. N., De Larco, J. E., and Todaro, G. J., Nerve growth factor receptors on human melanoma cells in culture, *Proc. Natl. Acad. Sci. U.S.A. 74*:565-569 (1977).

14. Pruss, R. M. and Herschman, H. R., Variants of 3T3 cells lacking mitogenic response to epidermal growth factor, *Proc. Natl. Acad. Sci., U.S.A. 74*:3918-3921 (1977).

15. Taylor, J. M., Cohen, S. and Mitchell, W. M., Epidermal growth factor: High and low molecular weight forms, *Proc. Natl. Acad. Sci., U.S.A. 67*:164-171 (1970).

16. Cohen, S., Taylor, J. M., Murakami, K., Michelakis, A. M. and Inagami, T., Isolation and characterization of renin-like enzymes from mouse submaxillary glands, *Biochemistry 11*:4286-4292 (1972).

17. Gospodarowicz, D., Greene, G. and Moran, J. S., Fibroblast growth factor can substitute for platelet factor to sustain the growth of BALB/3T3 cells in the presence of plasma, *Biochem. Biophys. Res. Commun. 65*:778-787 (1975).

18. Dulak, N. C. and Temin, H. M., A partially purified polypeptide fraction from rat liver cell conditioned medium with multiplication stimulating activity for embryo fibroblasts, *J. Cell Physiol. 81*:153-170 (1973).

19. Nissley, S. P. and Reekler, M. M., Multiplication-stimulating activity (MSA): A somatomedin-like polypeptide from cultured rat liver cells, *NCI Monograph:* The Association Research Conference, Lake Placid, New York, 1976, pp. 167-172.

20. De Larco, J. E. and Todaro, G. J., A human fibrosarcoma cell line producing multiplication stimulating activity (MSA)-rated peptides, *Nature 272*:356-358 (1978).

21. Levinson, A. D., Oppermann, H., Levintow, L., Jarmus, H. E. and Bishop, J. M., Evidence that the transforming gene of avian sarcoma virus encodes a protein kinase associated with a phosphotroein, *Cell 15*:561-572 (1978).

22. Collett, M. S. and Erikson, R. L., Protein kinase activity associated with the avian sarcoma virus src gene product, *Proc. Natl. Acad. Sci., U.S.A. 75*:2021-2024 (1978).

23. Sen, A., Todaro, G. J., Blair, D. G. and Robey, W. G., Thermolabile protein kinase molecules in a temperature-sensitive murine sarcoma virus pseudotype, *Proc. Natl. Acad. Sci., U.S.A. 76*: 3617-3621 (1979).

24. Sefton, B. M., Hunter, T., and Beemon, K., Temperature-sensitive transformation by Rous sarcoma virus temperature-sensitive protein kinase activity, *J. Virol. 33*:220-229 (1980).

INTERACTIONS OF MURINE LEUKEMIA VIRUSES WITH HEMATOPOIETIC STEM CELLS

Philip Furmanski
John Marcelletti
Candace S. Johnson

Department of Biology
Michigan Cancer Foundation
Detroit, Michigan

SUMMARY

Friend virus induces in susceptible mice an erythroblastic leukemia characterized by massive splenomegaly, hepatomegaly, viremia, and death. The RFV strain of Friend virus induces an initially identical disease, except that the leukemia spontaneously regresses in about 50% of the infected mice.

Leukemia regression is a macrophage-dependent process. Elimination or suppression of normal macrophage function with silica, carrageenan, antimacrophage serum, or trypan blue prevents regression. Macrophage phagocytic activity is inhibited in half of the leukemic mice at 25 days post virus-inoculation. Animals with macrophages that retain normal phagocytic function regress, whereas those with inhibited macrophage function do not. Progressor leukemic mice can be induced to regress by inoculation with normal, syngeneic macrophages.

Inhibition of macrophage function in leukemic progressor mice is the result of infection of macrophages with virus. Unstimulated, mature macrophages are refractory to infection with RFV or other strains of Friend virus. The resident, mature peritoneal macrophages in leukemic progressor mice become infected with virus as precursor bone marrow macrophage stem cells (CFU-C's). During RFV-induced leukemogenesis, the CFU-C's of all the mice become productively infected with the virus. In progressors, mature macrophages are produced which are infected and functionally inhibited. In regressor mice, the infected CFU-C's are eliminated and replaced with uninfected cells, which give rise to uninfected progeny capable of participating in or causing leukemia regression.

Thus, the outcome of the carcinogenic process initiated by Friend virus, an erythroleukemogenic agent, is determined by events which influence virus infection of other cellular compartments. Chemicals, growth factors or activators which affect cellular replication and virus infection of macrophage stem cells and their progeny will profoundly alter the course of the disease and its lethality.

Murine leukemia viruses (retroviruses) are presumed to cause leukemia by infection and transformation of particular pathognomonic hematopoietic stem cells [1,2]. But the progression of the leukemia, the development of its associated pathology, and its sequelae are unquestionably influenced by a variety of host factors which are also affected by the virus. These include immunological reactivity [3,4] and normal homeostatic mechanisms which regulate hematopoiesis [5,6]. An understanding of these functions could lead to new and effective methods for preventing, arresting, and reversing the neoplastic process.

Studies in our laboratory have focused on the identification and characterization of the host factors which influence leukemia. These studies make use of a model system which contrasts two initially identical leukemias: one in which the disease progresses and is ultimately lethal to the host; and one in which, following development of an indistinguishable acute leukemia, the disease spontaneously regresses and the animals return to a normal or near-normal state.

THE MODEL SYSTEM

The Friend murine leukemia virus (FV) induces, in susceptible mice,
a leukemia characterized by massive splenomegaly, hepatomegaly, viremia
and ultimately death in virtually all of the infected animals.

In 1969, Rich et al. [7,8] reported the isolation of a variant
of FV which induces a disease identical to that induced by the conventional strains of virus, but which spontaneously regresses in about
half the leukemic mice. In fully regressed animals, the spleen returns
to normal architecture and histology [9], virus is no longer detectable
in plasma or tissue extracts, and the mice exhibit a normal life span
[7,8]. The leukemias induced by FV and the variant, RFV, are histopathologically indistinguishable. Similarly, the leukemias induced
by RFV which will subsequently regress (regressors), and those which
will not (progressors), are histopathologically indistinguishable.

THE ROLE OF IMMUNOLOGICAL REACTIVITY IN LEUKEMIA REGRESSION

One of the primary host factors responsible for disease regression is
immunological reactivity. The leukemia induced by RFV does not regress
in animals in which immune functions have been suppressed by X-irradiation, neonatal thymectomy, congenital athymia, anti-thymocyte serum
treatment, or treatment with the bone-seeking isotope, ^{89}Sr [10,11].
In each case, regression is inhibited under conditions in which leukemogenesis is unaffected. Conversely, immunostimulation, using a
combination of specific (inactivated syngeneic leukemic cells) and
nonspecific (BCG) immunization, enhances leukemia regression [12].

Regressed mice exhibit potent immunological reactivity against
the virus and leukemia cells. Both humoral [13,14] and cell-mediated
[15] activities are detectable.

Sera from regressed mice possess complement-dependent and comple-
ment-independent neutralizing activity against the virus, and at least
two specificities of (complement-dependent) anti-leukemia cell cytotoxic antibodies. However, there is no association between the appear-

ance of these activities and subsequent disease regression, nor is
there any apparent correlation among the different humoral activities
detectable in sera from individual regressed mice.

In contrast, cell mediated immune reactivity against viral antigens and leukemia cells, measured using the agarose microdroplet assay
of macrophage migration inhibition, is detected in all regressed mice
[15]. Specific reactivity is also detectable in some leukemic mice,
and its presence is correlated with subsequent disease regression.

Other factors which influence leukemia regression are the genetic
composition of the host [16,17] and perturbations of the hematopoietic
system [18]. However, these factors have not yet been characterized,
and may affect regression through effects on the immune system.

MACROPHAGES AS EFFECTOR CELLS IN LEUKEMIA REGRESSION

Macrophages play a central role in regression of RFV-induced erythroleukemia [19,20]. This conclusion was derived from studies in which
macrophages were functionally eliminated from mice. Treatment of mice
with silica, carrageenan, trypan blue, or specific rabbit anti-mouse
macrophage sera inhibits regression (Table 1). The duration of the
effect on regression of each of these agents is related to their reported in vivo anti-macrophage effects. Additionally, poly (2-vinyl-
pyridine-N-oxide), which protects macrophages from the toxic effects
of silica and carrageenan, also inhibits their effects on regression
[19].

It is known that macrophage function, as measured by phagocytosis
of optimally opsonized sheep red blood cells, is depressed in FV-
infected leukemic mice [21,22]. We found that in RFV leukemic mice,
about 50% of the animals have macrophages with depressed phagocytic
activity, while the remainder have macrophages with normal or greater
than normal phagocytic function. All fully regressed mice have macrophages with normal phagocytic ability.

These results suggested a relationship between macrophage function and leukemia regression. To test this directly, small numbers

TABLE 1
Effects of Anti-Macrophage Agents on Leukemia Regression

	Treatment	Number of Leukemic Mice	% Regression[a]
Expt. 1	PBS	22	32
	PVNO	18	33
	Silica	20	0
	Carrageenan	19	5
	Trypan blue	20	5
	Silica + PVNO	20	30
	Carrageenan + PVNO	19	32
Expt. 2	PBS	10	60
	Anti-macrophage serum	15	0
	Pre-immune serum	14	64

[a]By day 46 post-virus inoculation

of peritoneal macrophages were removed from RFV-induced leukemic mice
and assayed for phagocytic ability. The animals were then monitored
for subsequent disease regression. We found that the phagocytic activity of the peritoneal macrophages is an extremely accurate prognos-
tic indicator for the course of the disease. The leukemia progressed
in those mice whose macrophages were inhibited, while in mice whose
macrophages remained normal, the disease regressed (Table 2).

The requirement for functionally competent macrophages for leukemia regression and the association between retention of macrophage
phagocytic activity in leukemic mice and subsequent disease regression
suggested that normal macrophages are responsible for the control and
reversal of the disease in RFV-infected animals. To test this hypothesis, FV-infected leukemic mice, which seldom regress, were inoculated
with normal syngeneic peritoneal macrophages [19,20]. This treatment
was effective in causing leukemia regression (Table 3). Treatment
with normal T-cells, nonadherent peritoneal wash cells, normal bone
marrow cells, or macrophages from progressor leukemic mice was ineffective.

TABLE 2
Leukemia Regression as a Function of Macrophage Phagocytic Activity

Phagocytic Activity	Number of Leukemic Mice Tested	Number Regressed
Normal[a]	24	22 (92%)[c]
Inhibited[b]	28	2 (7%)

[a] Phagocytic index $\geq$ 0.90.
[b] Phagocytic index $\leq$ 0.90.
[c] Percent regressed.

TABLE 3
Effect of Cell Transfer on FV Erythroleukemia

Treatment	Number Regressed/ Number Leukemic	% Regression
PBS	0/20	0
Normal macrophages	9/21	43
Leukemic macrophages	0/11	0
Normal bone marrow cells	0/9	0

INFECTION OF MACROPHAGES WITH FRIEND VIRUS

Previous studies have established that peritoneal macrophages become infected with the virus in mice inoculated with FV [21,23]. Peritoneal macrophages from mice with RFV-induced leukemia are also infected with virus. However, the proportion of infected cells in the macrophage population is directly related to the extent of inhibition of phagocytosis in these cells [19]. Macrophages isolated from regressor or regressed mice, which exhibit normal phagocytic activity, are rarely infected, as detected in the XC infectious center assay. Elimination of the infected macrophages from infected peritoneal cell populations, using cytotoxicity with anti-gp70 antibody and complement, restores the phagocytic index of the remaining cells to normal. Thus, macrophages from progressor mice are functionally inhibited and incapable of causing disease regression likely as a result of having been infected with virus.

Because resident peritoneal macrophages are mature differentiated cells which do not ordinarily synthesize DNA unless stimulated [24-26], and because productive infection with oncornaviruses requires DNA synthesis by the target cell [27-29], resident macrophages should be refractory to virus infection. However, infected macrophages are found in leukemic mice and appear to be a determinative factor in regression versus progression of the disease. It was important, therefore, to determine how the macrophages become infected in the progressor animals.

As reported by others, we found that resident peritoneal macrophages have undetectable or very low levels of DNA synthesis and do not become infected upon exposure to virus in vitro (Table 4). Cell transfer experiments showed that resident macrophages in leukemic progressor mice also do not become infected with virus in vivo [20]. In contrast, macrophages stimulated with either starch or thioglycollate in vivo, or colony stimulating factor (CSF) in vitro, exhibit much higher levels of DNA synthesis and are capable of being productively infected with virus in approximate proportion to their labeling indices (Table 4).

TABLE 4
Infection of Macrophages In Vitro with Friend Virus

	CSF	^{3}H-thymidine Incorporation	XC-Infectious Centers/10^5 Cells
Normal macrophages	-	46 ± 5[a]	0
	+	125 ± 20	1 ± 0.5
Exudate macrophages[b]	-	136 ± 3	6 ± 3
	+	$1,661 \pm 19$	40 ± 4

[a] cpm/10^5 macrophages, mean $\pm$ s.d.
[b] Starch induced.

These results suggested that infected macrophages in progressor mice must have become infected in a replicative phase of their development. During the process of differentiation from precursors in the bone marrow, the cells go through several divisions. We determined, therefore, whether macrophage precursors in the bone marrow could become infected with the virus. Bone marrow cells were exposed to virus in vitro and then placed in agar culture in the presence of L cell-derived CSF. Under these conditions, all the colonies obtained consisted of macrophages which had replicated and differentiated from their bone marrow precursors (CFU-C's). Six days later, the colonies were picked from the agar and tested for productive virus infection using the XC infectious center assay. In cultures of bone marrow cells initially exposed to virus approximately 50% of the resultant colonies were productively infected and consisted of infected, mature macrophages.

These results suggest that infection of CFU-C's in vivo could account for the differences in the peritoneal macrophage populations in regressor and progressor mice. Thus, in regressors, if the CFU-C compartment remained uninfected, progeny macrophages would also be uninfected, would remain functionally normal, and would thereby cause regression. In progressors, infected CFU-C's would give rise to infected macrophages incapable of causing regression.

TABLE 5
Infection of CFU-C's In Vivo

Days Post-Virus	Prognosis	Number of Mice	% Infected CFU-C's
14	Regression	4	100
	Progression	14	100
36	Regression	4	18[a]
	Progression	6	100

[a]Three mice had no infected CFU-C's; one had 75% infected CFU-C's.

To determine the relationship between infection of CFU-C's and leukemia regression, macrophages and bone marrow CFU-C's were removed from leukemic mice at 36 days post-virus inoculation, and tested for infection with virus. We found that the CFU-C's in the regressors (i.e., animals with uninfected mature peritoneal macrophages) were not productively infected with virus, while all CFU-C's from the progressors were infected. However, when assays were carried out on cells from mice at 15 days post-virus inoculation, all of the CFU-C's in both regressors and progressors were observed to be infected (Table 5).

Following inoculation with RFV, therefore, CFU-C's in all mice become infected, irrespective of whether the animals will subsequently regress. In the progressors, the infected CFU-C's give rise, ultimately, to functionally inhibited and infected macrophages. In the regressors, the infected CFU-C's are eliminated or replaced with uninfected CFU-C's.

Two mechanisms could account for these observations in the regressor mice. CFU-C's resistant to virus infection might arise and replace the susceptible CFU-C's in the regressors. Alternatively, regressor mice might be capable of eliminating CFU-C's which had become infected, leaving only the uninfected stem cells to populate the animal with mature macrophages. The latter mechanism could be accomplished by the potent immunological reactivity against viral antigens detectable in these mice [11-15].

These two possibilities can be distinguished by determining the susceptibility to virus infection of the CFU-C's in regressor mice. When these experiments were carried out, we found that CFU-C's from regressor mice are as susceptible to virus infection as are CFU-C's from normal animals. Therefore, infected CFU-C's in regressor mice must have been eliminated and replaced with uninfected cells.

The events which occur in the macrophage hematopoietic compartment following infection with RFV are schematically represented in Figure 1.

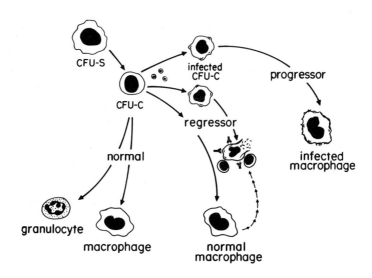

Figure 1. Schematic representation of the infection of macrophage precursors in leukemic progressor and regressor mice.

THE ROLE OF THE MACROPHAGE IN LEUKEMIA REGRESSION

The mechanisms by which macrophages influence the course of the leukemia induced by RFV are not known. Based on their almost ubiquitous
involvement in the development and manifestation of immunological
reactivity [30,31], especially in anti-tumor activity, and the requirement for an intact immune system in order for regression to occur, a
mechanism involving an immune effector function would not be unexpected. However, macrophages also play a significant role in regulation
of hematopoiesis [32,33]. Recent results obtained in our laboratory
support this function as a possible mechanism for the macrophage involvement in regression.

It has been shown that spleen erythropoietic precursor cells
CFU-E's) in mice inoculated with the polycythemia-inducing variant
of Friend virus are infected with virus and have lost their dependency
on the normal regulator of growth and maturation of erythroid cells,
erythropoietin [34,35]. Based on these and other studies, the CFU-E
or its direct precursor is considered to be the leukemic stem cell
of Friend disease [36].

However, we have found that in mice infected with RFV, CFU-E's
are neither erythropoietin independent, nor are they infected with
virus. Nonetheless, these animals develop typical Friend leukemias,
with massive splenomegaly, hepatomegaly, and large increases in the
numbers of erythroid precursors in splenic tissues. MacDonald et al.
[37] have reported that conventional anemia-producing strains of Friend
virus also do not induce erythropoietin-independent CFU-E's.

A possible mechanism for the pathology observed in Friend virus-
infected mice in the absence of abnormalities in the CFU-E compartment
is revealed by experiments on the interactions between macrophages
and erythropoietic precursors. Monolayers of normal macrophages inhibit colony formation by clonal agar cultures of normal CFU-E's Table
6). In contrast, monolayers of macrophages from leukemic progressor
mice (i.e. virus-infected macrophages) stimulate colony formation by
CFU-E's.

TABLE 6
Effect of Macrophages on CFU-E Colony Formation

Macrophag Macrophages	Number of Macrophages Added	CFU-E Colonies[a]
None	---	100
Normal	10^5	84
	10^4	102
	10^3	100
Leukemic	10^5	204
	10^4	145
	10^3	106

[a]Percent of control with no added macrophages.

These results suggest that infection of macrophages could, in the absence of other pathophysiological changes in the erythroid cells (i.e. erythropoietin-independence), be responsible for the enhanced erythropoiesis characteristic of the Friend virus-induced leukemias. Moreover, regression could occur because of the elimination of the infected macrophages, effectively removing the stimulus for overproduction of erythroid cells. This indirect mechanism for leukemogenesis and leukemia regression, and the specific relationships between virus infection of macrophages, stimulation of CFU-E's, and progression or regression of the disease, are currently under investigation.

CONCLUSIONS

The leukemia induced in mice with the RFV strain of Friend virus may either progress and kill the host, or spontaneously regress and pose no further threat to the life of the animal. Regressors are distinguished from progressors by their ability to eliminate virus-infected macrophage precursors. As a result, the regressors remain populated with normal, uninfected macrophages which are capable of causing leukemia regression. Macrophages may affect the course of the leukemia by participating in an effective immune response against the virus and leukemia cells. Infected macrophages in leukemic progressor mice may also be directly involved in the pathogenesis of the disease by stimulating proliferation of the apparent "stem cell" of the leukemia.

The studies carried out using this system have enabled us to identify and characterize host factors which can effectively modify the course of a leukemia. Studies are currently in progress to further define the specific mechanism(s) involved in these factors and to determine their applicability to other tumor - host systems.

ACKNOWLEDGMENTS

We thank Dr. Marvin A. Rich, whose encouragement and support have been invaluable to this work. These studies are supported by NIH grant CA-14100 and an Institutional Grant to the Michigan Cancer Foundation from the United Foundation of Detroit.

REFERENCES

1. Roussel, M., Soule, S., Lagrou, C., Rommens, C., Beug, H., Graf, T. and Stehelin, D., *Nature, 281*:452-455 (1979).

2. Kost, T. A., Koury, M. J., Hankins, W. D. and Krantz, S. B., *Cell, 18*:145-152 (1979).

3. Robinson, M. K., Manly, K. F. and Evans, M. J., *J. Immunol., 124*:1022-1027 (1980).

4. Klein, G. and Klein, E., *Proc. Natl. Acad. Sci., U.S.A., 74*:2121-2125 (1977).

5. Mirand, E., *National Cancer Institute Monograph No. 22,* pp. 482-502 (1966).

6. Marcelletti, J. and Furmanski, P., *Blood, 56*:134-137 (1980).

7. Rich, M. A., Siegler, R., Karl, S. and Clymer, R., *J. Natl. Cancer Inst., 42*:559-569 (1969).

8. Rich, M.A., Clymer, R. and Karl, S., *J. Natl. Cancer Inst., 42*: 571-577 (1969).

9. Russo, I., Russo, J., Baldwin, J. and Rich, M.A., *Am. J. Pathol., 85*:73-80 (1976).

10. Furmanski, P., Dietz, M., Fouchey, S., Hall, L., Clymer, R. and Rich, M. A., *J. Natl. Cancer Inst., 63*:449 (1979).

11. Dietz, M., Furmanski, P., Clymer, R. and Rich, M. A., *J. Natl. Cancer Inst., 57*:91-95 (1976).

12. Hines, D., Dietz, M., Rich, M. A. and Furmanski, P., *Cancer Immunol. Immunother., 5*:11-16 (1978).

13. Furmanski, P., Goodenow, R., Baldwin, J., Clymer, R. and Rich, M. A., *Fed. Proc., 34*:973 (1975).

14. Furmanski, P., Longley, C., Bolles, C. S., Hines, D. L. and Dietz, M., *J. Virology, 33*:1083 (1980).

15. Johnson, C. S., Fouchey, S. P. and Furmanski, P., *J. Natl. Cancer Inst., 64*:645-653 (1980).

16. Dietz, M. and Rich, M. A., *Int. J. Cancer, 10*:99-109 (1972).

17. Rich, M. A. and Dietz, M., *Proc. Soc. Exp. Biol., 137*:35-38 (1971).

18. Marcelletti, J. and Furmanski, P., unpublished observations.

19. Marcelletti, J. and Furmanski, P., *J. Immunol., 120*:1-8 (1979).

20. Marcelletti, J. and Furmanski, P., *Cell, 16*:649-659 (1979).

21. Levy, M. H. and Wheelock, E. F., *J. Reticuloendothelial Soc., 20*:243-254 (1976).

22. Wheelock, E. F., Caroline, N. L. and Moore, R. D., *J. Virol., 4*:1-6 (1969).

23. Levy, M. H. and Wheelock, E. F., *J. Immunol. 114*:962-965 (1975).

24. Dienstman, S. R. and Defendi, V., *Exp. Cell Res., 115*:191-199 (1973).

25. Stewart, C. C., Lin, H. and Adles, C., *J. Exp. Med., 141*:1114-1132 (1975).

26. van der Zeijst, B. A. M., Stewart, C. C. and Schlesinger, S., *J. Exp. Med., 147*:1253-1266 (1978).

27. Temin, H. M., *J. Cell Physiol., 69*:53-64 (1967).

28. Humphries, E. H. and Temin, H. M., *J. Virol., 14*:531-546 (1974).

29. Varmus, H. E., Padgett, T., Heasley, S., Simon, G. and Biship, S., *Cell, 11*:307-319 (1977).

30. Tzehoval, E., Segal, S. and Feldman, M., *Proc. Natl. Acad. Sci., U.S.A., 76*:4056-4060 (1979).

31. Beller, D. I. and Unanue, E. R., Role of Macrophages in the Regulation of Thymocyte Proliferation and Differentiation, in *Macrophage Regulation of Immunity* (E. R. Unanue and A. S. Rosenthal eds.), Academic Press, New York, 1980, pp. 361-378.

32. Kurland, J. I., Meyers, P. A. and Moore, M. A. S., *J. Exp. Med., 151*:839-852 (1980).

33. Shaklai, M. and Tavassoli, M., *J. Ultrastructural Research, 69*: 343-361 (1979).

34. McGarry, M. P. and Mirand, E. A., *Exp. Hemat., 1*:174-182 (1973).

35. Liao, S.-K. and Axelrad, A. A., *Int. J. Cancer, 15*:467-482 (1975).

36. Opitz, U. and Seidel, H.-J., *Blut, 37*:183-192 (1978).

MECHANISMS IN CHEMICAL CARCINOGENESIS

ACTIVATION OF CARCINOGENIC POLYCYCLIC HYDROCARBONS BY METABOLISM

Philip L. Grover

Chester Beatty Research Institute
Institute of Cancer Research
Royal Cancer Hospital
London, United Kingdom

INTRODUCTION

The polycyclic hydrocarbons are of interest as carcinogens because their presence in the environment [1] is thought to be associated with an increased incidence of cancer of several sites in man. Members of this class of chemical carcinogens are commonly formed as products of the incomplete combustion of organic materials [2] and they are therefore relatively inert compounds that are lipophilic and show only slight solubility in water. Structurally, they are composed of fused benzene rings that may or may not be substituted with alkyl groups (Figure 1). The arrangement of the benzene rings and the sites of substitution have a marked effect on carcinogenic potency [3]; for example, the addition of methyl groups to the 7- and 12-positions of benz(a)anthracene converts a weak carcinogen into a highly active compound.

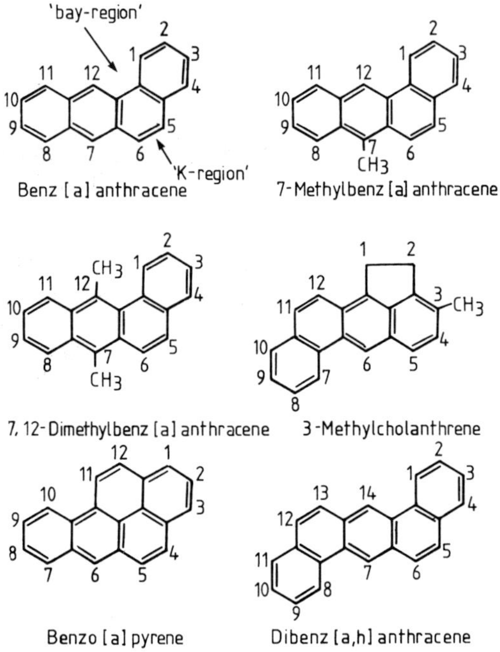

Figure 1. Structural formulae of carcinogenic polycyclic hydrocarbons.

Terrestrial species must metabolize the polycyclic hydrocarbons with which they become contaminated in order to excrete them, and hydroxylation reactions predominate in the conversion of hydrocarbons to more polar derivatives [4]. Many hydroxylated derivatives then become conjugated with, for example, glucuronic or sulphuric acid, which increases their water solubility still further. The enzymes involved in the metabolism of the hydrocarbons are the battery of drug-metabolizing enzymes that are widely distributed within the animal kingdom, and it is in the metabolism of the polycyclic hydrocarbons that "mistakes" occur that lead, in some cases, to the formation of metabolites that are more, rather than less, hazardous to the organism.

HYDROCARBON METABOLISM

It has been known for many years that the first stage in the metabolism of a typical polycyclic hydrocarbon is usually the addition of
one atom of oxygen across an aromatic double bond, a type of reaction
catalysed by the NADPH-dependent mono-oxygenases that are present
predominantly in the endoplasmic reticulum of cells [5]. The simple
epoxide so formed can then either (a) rearrange, non-enzymically, to
the corresponding phenol, (b) be hydrated, by the addition of one
molecule of water, to yield a dihydrodiol, a reaction catalysed by
epoxide hydratase [6] that is also predominantly microsomal, or (c)
be conjugated with the tripeptide glutathione, a type of reaction catalysed by the soluble glutathione S-transferases [7] (Figure 2). This
latter reaction leads ultimately to the formation of acetylcysteine
derivatives that are excreted in urine and are known as mercapturic
acids.

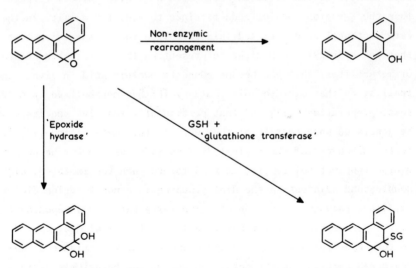

Figure 2. Further metabolism of a simple K-region epoxide to the corresponding phenol, dihydrodiol and glutathione conjugate.

Simple epoxides, especially those of the K-region type, were strongly suspected for some time of being the reactive species, or "ultimate carcinogens" [8], formed from the hydrocarbons since they possessed many of the chemical and biological properties that were thought to be relevant [4]. Thus they were alkylating agents that would react covalently with nucleic acids either present in solution or in cells in culture, they were mutagenic in several test systems, and they were capable of inducing the malignant transformation of cultured mammalian cells: when tested for carcinogenicity they were, however, almost always less active than their parent hydrocarbons.

The "K-region epoxide hypothesis" had to be abandoned when it was clearly shown, using Sephadex LH20 column chromatography, that the hydrocarbon-nucleic acid adducts formed in cells or in tissues treated with a polycyclic hydrocarbon were not the same as the adducts that were formed when the related K-region epoxide reacted with nucleic acids [9,10]. These studies also showed that the hydrocarbon-nucleic acid adducts formed following metabolic activation were more polar than the K-region epoxide adducts since they eluted earlier in the water-methanol gradient, and this gave rise to the suspicion that more than one hydroxyl group might be present on the hydrocarbon metabolite, or metabolites, that had become bound to nucleic acid in vivo. The realization that dihydrodiols could be further metabolized in microsomal preparations [11] and that particularly reactive species could be generated when certain of them were further metabolized [12] led to the discovery of the vicinal diol-epoxides as a new type polycyclic hydrocarbon metabolite [13] that is formed when the isolated, olefinic double bond adjacent to the diol grouping in a non-K-region diol is oxidized, through the action of a mono-oxygenase, to an epoxide (Figure 3). For some time the further metabolism of vicinal diol-epoxides to tetrahydrotetrols and to glutathione conjugates (Figure 3) was neglected partly, one suspects, because of the relatively rapid solvolysis that occurs with the most popular benzo(a)pyrene derivatives. It has now been shown, however, that diol-epoxides, like the anti-8,9-diol 10,11-oxide of benz(a)anthracene and the anti-7,8-diol 9,10-oxide of benzo(a)pyrene, do form glutathione conjugates in enzyme-

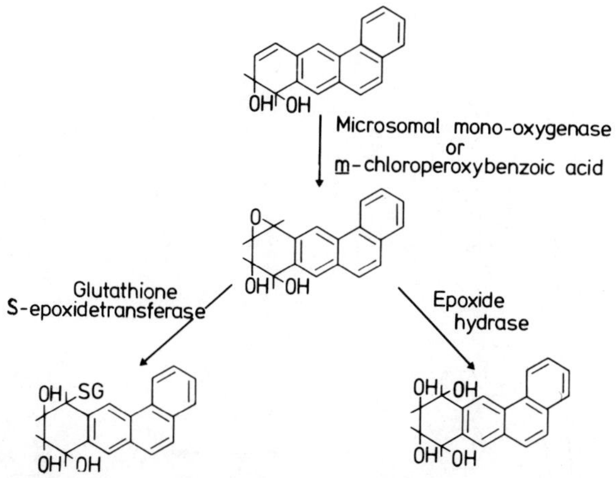

Figure 3. Formation and further metabolism of a vicinal diol-epoxide, 8,9-dihydro-8,9-dihydroxybenz(a)anthracene 10,11-oxide.

catalysed reactions [14,15], and the role of epoxide hydrase in cata-
lysing the conversion of diol-epoxides to tetrahydrotetrols is under
close examination [16]. Such studies are of interest because metabolism that leads to the removal of potentially-reactive intermediates
may be just as important as the reactions leading to their formation.
The discovery of the diol-epoxides led in turn to a great deal of
work on (a) the possibility that the formation of vicinal diol-epoxides
might prove to be a general mechanism for the metabolic activation of
the polycyclic hydrocarbons as a class of chemical carcinogens and
on (b) the identification of the particular diol-epoxides most likely
to be responsible for the biological effects of individual hydrocarbons.

DIOL-EPOXIDES AS REACTIVE INTERMEDIATES

Some of the progress that has been made, as well as some of the problems and pitfalls that have been encountered, in attempting to obtain
evidence pertaining to the areas referred to in (a) and (b) above will
now be discussed.

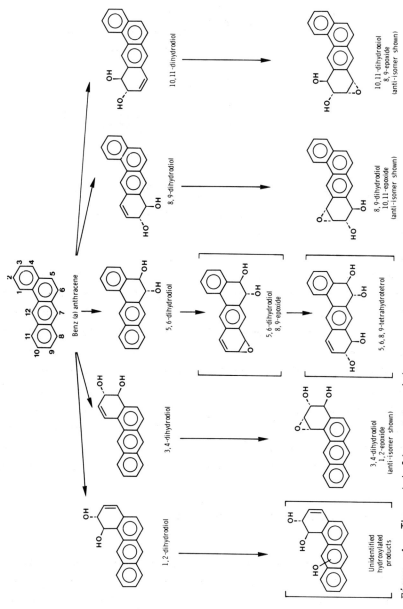

Figure 4. The metabolism of benz(a)anthracene to diols and diol-epoxides.

With benz(a)anthracene, for example, five trans-dihydrodiols are
possible (Figure 4) (metabolically-formed dihydrodiols usually possess
the trans-configuration, see Ref. 4) and the metabolites formed from
benz(a)anthracene by rat liver preparations appear to include all five
possible trans-diols [17]. In addition, both the 3,4- and 8,9-dihydro-
diols appear to be formed by mouse skin maintained in short-term organ
culture [18] and by hamster embryo cells [19]. Only four of these
five diols can form vicinal diol-epoxides since the K-region diol,
the 5,6-diol, lacks an olefinic double bond adjacent to the dihydrodiol group; a non-vicinal diol-epoxide is possible in theory (Figure
4), but this has not been detected. The metabolic conversion of dihydrodiols to diol-epoxides appears to be markedly affected by diol
conformation: diols normally adopt the preffered quasi-diequatorial
conformation but, if the diol groups are adjacent to a "bay" in the
molecule or to an alkyl substituent, they may be forced to adopt a
quasi-diaxial conformation (Figure 5). Incidentally, diol conformation

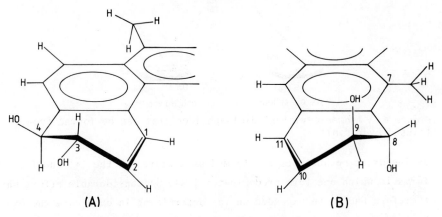

(A)   (B)

Figure 5. Conformations adopted by dihydrodiols. A. Quasi-diequatorial conformation adopted by unhindered dihydrodiols. B. Quasi-
diaxial conformation adopted by dihydrodiols that are formed, for
example, in proximity to an alkyl substituent or in a "bay-region".

is also known to have a marked effect on the chromatographic properties
of diols [20,21]. One of the four non-K-region dihydrodiols that can
be formed from benz(a)anthracene, the "bay-region" 1,2-diol, exists
in a predominantly quasi-diaxial conformation [22] and does not appear

to be converted to a diol-epoxide, possibly because stereochemical
effects prevent it from acting as a substrate for monooxygenases.
The other three non-K-region diols can each be converted to vicinal
diol-epoxides (Figure 4), and from early work on benzo(a)pyrene activation, it is known that each dihydrodiol can give rise to two sterio-
isomeric diol-epoxides (Figure 6), the syn in which the benzylic hydroxyl group is on the same face of the ring as the epoxide moiety
and the anti, in which it is on the opposite face of the ring. The
two forms show appreciably different rates of reaction with, for example, nucleic acids as predicted [23], and also differing stabilities.

A further complication concerns the existence of enantiomeric,
or optically-active, forms of diols and diol-epoxides. Since they
are formed by enzyme-catalysed reactions that are certainly stereo-
selective even if they are not completely stereo-specific, diol and

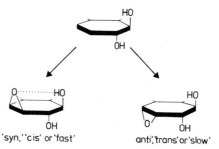

Figure 6. Isomeric vicinal diol-epoxides that can be formed from a
trans-dihydrodiol.

diol-epoxide metabolites are formed as mixtures of the (+) and (-)
forms in which one form predominates [24]. A considerable effort has
therefore had to be expended on (a) determining in each case the extent of the optical purity of products isolated from metabolism experiments and (b) resolving the racemic mixtures that are obtained
by synthesis into their optically-active forms [25]. Studies in this
area may well be very relevant to hydrocarbon activation, since the
two enantiomeric forms of one diol-epoxide have been found to differ
markedly in their reactivity towards nucleic acid [26] and in their
biological activities [27].

As far as the involvement of diol-epoxides in the metabolic activation of benz(a)anthracene is concerned, the hydrocarbon can be activated, in theory, through the formation of vicinal diol-epoxides in either the 1,2,3.4- or the 8,9,10,11-rings. Recent fluorescence spectral evidence [28] indicates that the principal metabolites that react with nucleic acids in mouse skin or in hamster embryo cells treated with benz(a)anthracene possess an intact phenanthrene nucleus which is consistent with activation involving diol-epoxide formation in the 8,9,10,11-ring, as suggested originally [29]. Chromatographic examination of the hydrocarbon-deoxyribonucleoside adducts that are formed when benz(a)anthracene is metabolized by microsomes in the presence of DNA [30] or by hamster embryo cells in culture [31] or when benz(a)anthracene is applied to mouse skin in vivo [32] has confirmed this, and has indicated that the anti-isomer of the 8,9-diol 10,11-oxide is the principal reactive species concerned, although variable amounts of adducts arising from the anti 3,4-diol 1,2-oxide are also present in DNA isolated from these different systems. Interestingly, the 8,9-diol 10,11-oxide of benz(a)anthracene (Figure 3) was the first vicinal diol-epoxide to be detected as a metabolite of a dihydrodiol [13], and chromatographic comparisons with synthetic dio diol-epoxides indicate that it is the anti-isomer that is formed enzymically [33]. Additional evidence indicates that the main site of reaction of the anti 8,9-diol 10,11-oxide is with the extranuclear amino groups of guanine residues [34], although some reaction with adenosine has also been detected: one of the principal 8,9-diol 10,11-oxide-guanosine adducts has also been characterized [35] and its structure is shown in Figure 7.

In contrast to the data cited above, indicating the involvement of the 8,9-diol 10,11-oxide in the metabolic activation of benz(a) anthracene, the results of tests for biological activity have suggested that the most active diol-epoxides are the 3,4-diol 1,2-oxides. The 3,4-diol and the related syn and anti 3,4-diol 1,2-oxides were much more potent as mutagens in S. typhimurium or in V79 Chinese hamster cells [36-39] and as carcinogens on mouse skin [38,40,41] or in new-

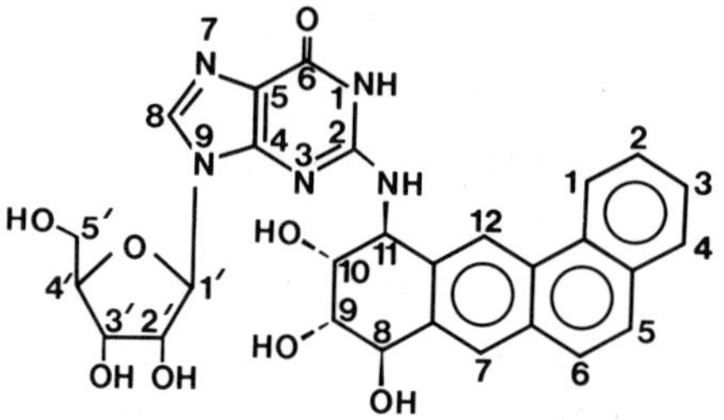

Figure 7. Structure of a benz(a)anthracene-guanosine adduct formed through the reaction of the ring opened form of the anti 8,9-diol 10,11-oxide of benz(a)anthracene with the exocyclic amino group of guanosine.

born mice [42] than other metabolites that were tested, although the 3,4-diol did fail to induce malignant transformation of cultured mammalian cells [39].

This particular paradox highlights the problems now being experienced by those attempting to apply the "bay-region" theory to hydrocarbon activation. On the basis of a series of perturbational molecular orbital calculations, it was originally predicted that carbonium ions could be formed more readily from an epoxide that is adjacent to a "bay" in a hydrocarbon molecule, that is the region formed by an angular benzene ring (Figure 1), than from any other non-"bay-region" epoxide [43]. These predictions, which have become embodied in the "bay-region" theory, mean that diol-epoxides like those shown in Figure 8 should be the most chemically-reactive epoxides that can be formed from these particular hydrocarbons. For the potent carcinogens like benzo(a)pyrene, 3-methylcholanthrene, 7-methylbenz(a)anthracene, 7,12-dimethylbenz(a)anthracene, and dibenz(a,h)anthracene, the available evidence on metabolic activation, obtained from a variety of different experimental approaches, supports these predictions. The most chemically-reactive diol-epoxides, i.e. those of the "bay-region" type, also seem to be those that are involved in the mediation of biological activities such as mutagenesis and tumour-initiation and in reactions with nucleic acids in vivo. As a means of predicting the reactivity of diol-epoxides, the bay-region hypothesis has therefore been most valuable, but it has not been successfully extrapolated into a "bay-region theory of polycyclic aromatic hydrocarbon carcinogenesis" re-

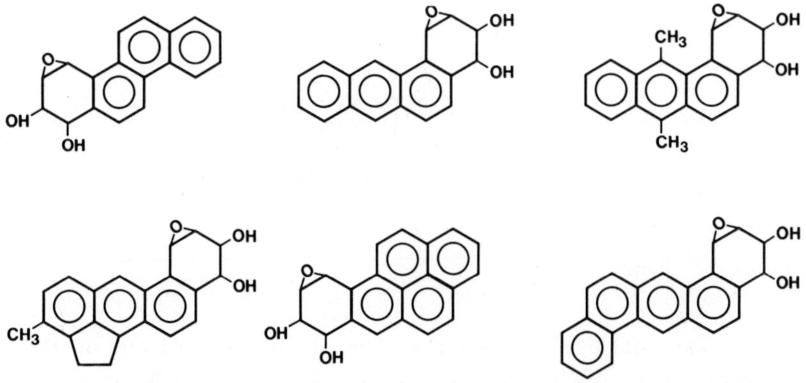

Figure 8. Reactive "bay-region" diol-epoxides of chrysene, benz(a)
anthracene, 7,12-dimethylbenz(a)anthracene, 3-methylcholanthrene,
benzo(a)pyrene and dibenz(a,h)anthracene.

gardless of suggestions to the contrary [42,44-46]. There are, in
addition to epoxide reactivity, a variety of other factors, many of
which are not yet well understood, that will have to be taken in
account before the carcinogenic potency of a novel hydrocarbon, and
the mechanism by which it is activated by metabolism, can be predicted
from its structure. In such a case, the formation of a particular
vicinal diol-epoxide may be suspected of being important but, without
actual information on the metabolism of the hydrocarbon and preferably
that which occurs in a target tissue, it is impossible to say whether
a reactive diol-epoxide is formed or not. Taking benzo(e)pyrene (Figure 9) as an example, calculations predict that the "bay-region" diol-
epoxides, the 9,10-diol 10,11-oxide, should be reactive [43]: the
hydrocarbon itself lacks carcinogenicity presumably because (a) the
precursor diol, the 9,10-diol, is not formed as a metabolite to any
appreciable extent [47] and (b) even if the diol was formed, its further metabolism does not appear to yield the diol-epoxide [48]. On
the basis of the "bay-region" theory as originally proposed, and without this information on metabolism, the hydrocarbon would have been
predicted to be carcinogenic. The same sort of situation seems likely to pertain in the case of dibenz(a,c)anthracene, another weakly-
active or inactive hydrocarbon where considerably less information
is available as yet.

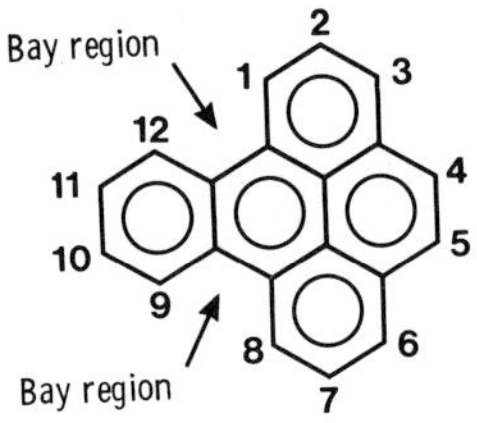

Figure 9. Benzo(e)pyrene

It was quite fortuitous that benzo(a)pyrene was one of the first compounds whose metabolic activation was examined from the point of view of diol-epoxide formation [49], since it has actually turned out to be one of the simpler situations studies. Very considerable progress has been made with this most popular hydrocarbon which is activated through the formation of the 7,8-diol 9,10-oxide (Figure 8), and much of the data have been reviewed [50]. Figure 10 shows, for example, the structure of the adduct in which the carbonium ion formed at C_{10} of the hydrocarbon by epoxide ring opening has reacted with the exocyclic amino group of deoxyguanosine. A lot of the information obtained with benzo(a)pyrene is now being applied in studies on the activation of other hydrocarbons.

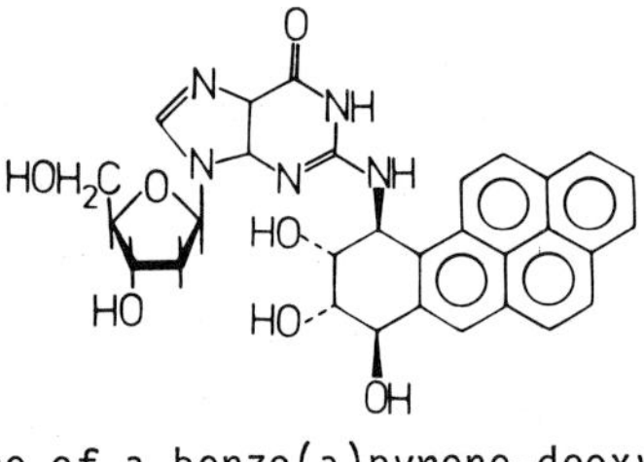

Figure 10. Structure of a benzo(a)pyrene-deoxyguanosine adduct formed through reaction of the ring-opened form of the anti 7,8-diol 9,10-oxide of benzo(a)pyrene with the exocyclic amino group of deoxygranosine.

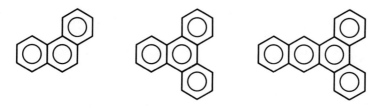

Figure 11. Inactive or very weakly active hydrocarbons possessing "bay-regions". From left to right phenanthrene, triphenylene and dibenz(a,c)anthracene.

As noted above, the "bay-region" theory of epoxide reactivity, as it might well be called, has been successful in predicting the diol-epoxides that are apparently involved in the activation of some of the hydrocarbons that are potent carcinogens. However, it does not appear to apply to others like benz(a)anthracene. It ought also to be borne in mind (a) that the possession of a "bay-region" does not of itself confer carcinogenicity upon a compound (Figure 11) and (b) that, conversely, the absence of a "bay-region" does not automatically result in an inactive compound (Figure 12) since exceptions to both generalizations are well known. In the widest sense, the formation of non-K-region diol metabolites may be of importance in terms of activation solely because they provide a source of olefinic double bonds in a class of compounds that are normally fully unsaturated. If the dihydrodiol grouping is permitted by its stereochemical environment to adopt the preferred quasi-diequatorial conformation, then the olefinic double bonds adjacent to the diol grouping may be metabolized to vicinal diol-epoxides by mono-oxygenases. If these diol-epoxides are not good substrates for further metabolism to tetrols or to conjugates, if the right enantiomer predominates, and if the epoxide group can ring open with sufficient ease to yield a reactive benzylic carbonium ion, then covalent reactions with, for example, cellular macromolecules may occur.

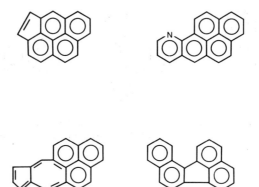

Figure 12.   Carcinogenic compounds that lack "bay-regions".

HYDROCARBON CARCINOGENESIS

Although there are now fair amounts of data on the reactivities of
various diol-epoxides towards nucleic acids (i.e. refs. 34, 51, 52),
there is no clear explanation as yet for the marked variations in
carcinogenic potency of the parent hydrocarbons and, in addition, not
nearly enough is known about the biological effectiveness of the different types of hydrocarbon-nucleic acid adducts that are now being
identified and characterized.   It has been claimed that the extents
of covalent reaction with adenine that occur when polycyclic hydrocarbons are metabolized correlates with the carcinogenicities of the
hydrocarbons [53], but the system used was somewhat artificial.   There
has also been a report that the extents of reaction with DNA that
occur in the skin when mice of three strains showing different suscep-
tibilities to hydrocarbon carcinogenesis are treated with 7,12-
dimethylbenz(a)anthracene are the same [54].   This also requires con-
firmation since it could have an important bearing on the relevance
of overall extents of reaction with DNA to hydrocarbon carcinogenesis:
the rapid disappearance of some adducts by an error-prone repair mechanism could conceivably be of more importance than the detectable per-
sistence of others.

When the data cited on the metabolic activation of polycyclic hydrocarbons are considered, it is apparent that a general picture of the metabolic mechanisms of hydrocarbon activation is now being rapidly built up. What seems likely to be the most difficult phase of research on hydrocarbon carcinogenesis has yet to begin in earnest, however. Whilst nucleic acids are still very strongly suspected of being the important intracellular targets for reactive hydrocarbon metabolites, the correlations between DNA reaction and hydrocarbon carcinogenicity could be coincidental rather than causal, with the nucleic acids acting as nucleophilic trapping agents. Even if some of the reactions of hydrocarbon metabolites with the nucleic acids are shown to be causally related to carcinogenesis, explanations of precisely how this occurs and how it might be prevented will still have to be sought. It is also in this area of mechanisms that the most fruitful collaboration between those working on the modes of action of, say, radiation, tumour viruses, and/or chemical carcinogens seems likely to occur. Agents as diverse as these are all able to bring about the malignant transformation of cells and, since their effects, i.e. the induction of malignancy, are so similar, there must be a strong suspicion that the mechanisms involved in the process are, at the very least, convergent if they are not actually identical.

REFERENCES

1. Committee on Biologic Effects of Atmospheric Pollutants, Particulate Polycyclic Organic Matter, *Natl. Acad. Sci.*, Washington D.C., 1972.

2. Guerin, M. R., Epler, J. L., Griest, W. H., Clark, B. R. and Rao, T. K., Polycyclic aromatic hydrocarbons from fossil fuel conversion processes. In: Carcinogenesis, Vol. 3. (P. W. Jones and R. I. Freudenthal, eds.) *Raven Press,* New York, 1978, pp. 21-33.

3. Dipple, A., Polynuclear Aromatic Hydrocarbons. In: ACS Monograph Series No. 173 (C. E. Searle, ed.), *American Chemical Society,* 1976, pp. 245-314.

4. Sims, P. and Grover, P. L., *Adv. Cancer Res., 20:*165-274 (1974).

5. Esterbrook, R. W. and Lindenlamb, E., The Induction of Drug Metabolims. Symposia Medica Hoechst No. 14, *Stuttgart:Schattauer Verlag,* 1979.

6. Oesch, F., *Xenobiotica, 3:*305-340 (1973).

7. Chasseaud, L. F., *Adv. Cancer Res., 29:*176-275 (1979).

8. Miller, J. A., *Cancer Res., 30:*559-576 (1970).

9. Baird, W. M., Dipple, A., Gover, P. L., Sims, P. and Brookes, P., *Cancer Res., 33:*2386-2392 (1973).

10. Baird, W. M., Harvey, R. G. and Brookes, P., *Cancer Res., 35:*54-57 (1975).

11. Booth, J., Keysell, G. R. and Sims, P., *Biochem. Pharmacol., 22:* 1781-1791 (1973).

12. Borgen, A., Darvey, H., Castagnoli, N., Crocker, T. T., Rasmussen, R. E. and Yang, I. Y., *J. Med. Chem., 16:*502-506 (1963).

13. Booth, J. and Sims, P., *FEBS Lett., 47:*30-33 (1974).

14. Cooper, C. S., Hewer, A., Ribeiro, O., Grover, P. L. and Sims, P., *FEBS Lett., 118:*39-42 (1980).

15. Cooper, C. S., Hewer, A., Ribeiro, O., Grover, P. L. and Sims, P., *Carcinogenesis, 1:*1075-1080 (1980).

16. Glatt, H. R. and Oesch, F., personal communication.

17. Tierney, B., Hewer, A., MacNicoll, A. D., Gervasi, P. G., Rattle, H., Walsh, C., Gover, P. L. and Sims, P., *Chem.-Biol. Interactions, 23:*243-257 (1978).

18. MacNicoll, A. D., Grover, P. L. and Sims, P., *Chem.-Biol. Interactions, 29:*169-188 (1980).

19. MacNicoll, A. D., Cooper, C. S., Ribeiro, O., Grover, P. L. and Sims, P., *Proc. Am. Ass. Cancer Res., 21:*70 (1980).

20. Thakker, D. R., Yagi, H. and Jerina, D. M., *Methods Enzymol., 52C:*279-296 (1978).

21. Tierney, B., Burden, P., Hewer, A., Ribeiro, O., Walsh, C., Rattle, H., Grover, P. L. and Sims, P., *J. Chromatog., 176:*329-335 (1979).

22. Jerina, D. M., Selander, H., Yagi, H., Wells, M. C., Davey, J. F., Mahedevan, V. and Gibson, D. T., *J. Amer. Chem. Soc., 98:*5988-5996 (1976).

23. Hulbert, P. B., *Nature (London) 256*:146-148 (1975).

24. Thakker, D. R., Levin, W., Yagi, H., Turujman, S., Kapadia, D., Conney, A. H. and Jerina, D. M., *Chem.-Biol. Interactions, 27*:145-161 (1979).

25. Levin, W., Thakker, D. R., Wood, A. W., Chang, R. L., Lehr, R. E., Jerina, D. M. and Conney, A. H., *Cancer Res., 38*:1705-1710 (1978).

26. Pulkrabek, P., Leffler, S., Grunberger, D. and Weinstein, I. B., *Biochemistry, 18*:5128-5134 (1979).

27. Buening, M. K., Wislocki, P. G., Levin, W., Yagi, H., Thakker, D. R., Akagi, H., Koreeda, M., Jerina, D. M. and Conney, A. H., *Proc. Natl. Acad. Sci., U.S.A., 75*:5358-5361 (1978).

28. Vigny, P., Kindts, M., Duquesne, M., Cooper, C. S., Grover, P. L. and Sims, P., *Carcinogenesis, 1*:33-36 (1980).

29. Swaisland, A. J., Hewer, A., Pal, K., Keysell, G. R., Booth, J., Grover, P. L. and Sims, P., *FEBS Lett., 47*:34-39 (1974).

30. MacNicoll, A. D., Cooper, C. S., Ribeiro, O., Gervasi, P. G., Hewer, A., Walsh, C., Grover, P. L. and Sims, P., *Biochem. Biophys. Res. Commun., 91*:490-497 (1979).

31. Cooper, C. S., MacNicoll, A. D., Ribeiro, O., Gervasi, P. G., Hewer, A., Walsh, C., Pal, K., Grover, P. L. and Sims, P., *Cancer Lett., 9*:53-59 (1980).

32. Cooper, C. S., Ribeiro, O., Hewer, A., Walsh, C., Pal, K., Grover, P. L. and Sims, P., *Carcinogenesis, 1*:233-243 (1980).

33. Sims, P. and Grover, P. L., *Med. Biol. Environ., 4*:315-329 (1976).

34. Hemminki, K., Cooper, C. S., Ribeiro, O., Grover, P. L. and Sims P., *Carcinogenesis 1*:277-286 (1980).

35. Cary, P. D., Turner, C. H., Cooper, C. S., Ribeiro, O., Grover, P. L. and Sims, P., *Carcinogenesis, 1*:505-512 (1980).

36. Wood, A. W., Levin, W., Lu, A. Y. H., Ryan, D., West, S. B., Lehr, R. E., Schaefer-Ridder, M., Jerina, D. M. and Conney, A. H., *Biochem. Biophys. Res. Commun., 72*:680-686 (1976).

37. Wood, A. W., Chang, R. L., Levin, W., Lehr, R. E., Schaefer-Ridder, M., Karle, J. M., Jerina, D. M. and Conney, A. H., *Proc. Natl. Acad. Sci., U.S.A., 74*:2746-2750 (1977).

38. Slaga, T. J., Huberman, E., Selkirk, J. K., Harvey, R. G., and Bracken, W. M., *Cancer Res., 38*:1699-1704 (1978).

39. Marquardt, H., Baker, S., Tierney, B., Grover, P. L. and Sims, P., *Brit. J. Cancer, 39*:540-547 (1979).

40. Wood, A. W., Levin, W., Chang, R. L., Lehr, R. E., Schaefer-Ridder, M., Karle, J. M., Jerina, D. M. and Conney, A. H., *Proc. Natl. Acad. Sci., U.S.A., 74*:3176-3179 (1977).

41. Levin, W., Thakker, D. R., Wood, A. W., Chang, R. L., Lehr, R. E., Jerina, D. M. and Conney, A. H., *Cancer Res., 38*:1705-1710 (1978).

42. Wislocki, P. G., Kapitulnik, J., Levin, W., Lehr, R. E., Schaefer-Ridder, M., Karle, J. M., Jerina, D. M. and Conney, A. H., *Cancer Res., 38*:693-696 (1978).

43. Jerina, D. M. and Lehr, R. E., The Bay-Region Theory: a Quantum Mechanical Approach to Aromatic Hydrocarbon-induced Carcinogenicity. In: Microsomes and Frug Oxidation (V. Ullrich, I. Roots, A. G. Hilderbrandt, R. W. Estabrook and A. H. Conney, eds.), *Pergamon Press, Oxford U. K.,* 1977, pp. 709-720.

44. Wood, A. W., Chang, R. L., Levin, W., Lehr, R. E., Schaefer-Ridder, M., Karle, J. M., Jerina, D. M. and Conney, A. H., *Proc. Natl. Acad. Sci., U.S.A., 74*:2746-2750 (1977).

45. Levin, W., Buening, M. K., Wood, A. W., Chang, R. L., Thakker, D. R., Jerina, D. M. and Conney, A. H., *Cancer Res., 39*:3549-3553 (1979).

46. Buening, M. K., Levin, W., Wood, A. W., Chang, R. L., Lehr, R. E., Taylor, C. W., Yagi, H., Jerina, D. M. and Conney, A. H., *Cancer Res., 40*:203-206 (1980).

47. MacLeod, M. C., Cohen, G. M. and Selkirk, J. K., *Cancer Res., 39*:3463-3470 (1979).

48. Levin, W., Wood, A. W., Buening, M. K., Kumar, S., Lehr, R. E., Jerina, D. M. and Conney, A. H., *Proc. Am. Ass. Cancer Res., 20*:222 (1979).

49. Sims, P., Grover, P. L., Swaisland, A., Pal, K. and Hewer, A., *Nature (London), 252*:326-328 (1974).

50. Gelboin, H. V. and Ts'o, P. O. P. eds. Polycyclic Hydrocarbons and Cancer, *Academic Press, New York,* 1978.

51. Phillips, D. H., Grover, P. L. and Sims, P., *Chem.-Biol. Interactions, 20*:63-75 (1978).

52. Hsu, W. T., Lin, E. J., Fu, P. P., Harvey, R. G. and Weiss, S. B., *Biochem. Biophys. Res. Commun., 88*:251-257 (1979).

53. DiGiovanni, J., Romson, J. R., Linville, D., Juchau, M. R. and
     Slaga, R. J., *Cancer Lett.*, 7:39-43 (1979).

54. Phillips, D. H., Grover, P. L. and Sims, P., *Int. J. Cancer,*
     22:487-494 (1979).

MULTISTAGE SKIN TUMOR PROMOTION:
INVOLVEMENT OF A PROTEIN KINASE

Mark Mamrack
Thomas J. Slaga

Biology Division
Oak Ridge National Laboratory
Oak Ridge, Tennessee

INTRODUCTION

Current information suggests that chemical carcinogenesis is a multi-
step process with one of the best studied models in this regard being
the two-stage carcinogenesis system using mouse skin. Skin tumors
can be induced by the sequential application of a subthreshold dose
of a carcinogen (initiation phase) followed by repetitive treatment
with a noncarcinogenic tumor promoter. The initiation phase requires
only a single application of either a direct or indirect carcinogen
at a subthreshold dose and is essentially irreversible; the promotion
phase is brought about by repetitive treatments after initiation and
is initially reversible, later becoming irreversible.

TABLE 1
Dose-Response Studies on the Ability of TPA
to Promote Tumors After DMBA Initiation[a]

Promoter	Dose (ug)	Time to First Papillima (wks)	# of Papillomas per Mouse at 15 Weeks	With Papillomas at 15 Weeks	With Carcinomas at 50 Weeks
TPA	10	8	3.0	100	32
TPA	5	6	7.2	100	46
TPA	2	7	6.5	100	45
TPA	1	8	3.6	80	25
TPA	0.1	11	0.4	5	8

[a]The mice were initiated with 10 nmoles of DMBA and promoted one week later with various dose levels of TPA.

The dose-response ability of 12-0-tetradecanoylphorbol-13-acetate
(TPA) to promote tumors after DMBA initiation is shown in Table 1.
There is a very good dose-response relationship for tumor promotion
when considering either the number of papillomas per mouse at 15 weeks
or the percent of mice with squamous cell carcinomas at 50 weeks.
Similar results have been reported using Charles River CD-1 mice [1,2]
or ICR/Ha Swiss mice [3,4]. The repetitive application of the promoter TPA without initiation generally produces very few tumors but
not in a dose-dependent manner [1,4].

Recently, the generality of the two-stage system or multistage
carcinogenesis has been shown to exist in a number of systems besides
the skin such as the liver, bladder, colon, esophagus, stomach, mammary, diaplacental as well as cells in culture [5]. Various two-stage
systems with the initiating and promoting agents involved are shown
in Table 2. It is apparent that quite a diversity of initiating and
promoting agents exists among the various two-stage systems.

Tumor Initiation

The tumor initiation phase appears to be an irreversible step which
probably involves a somatic cell mutation as evidenced by the correlation between the carcinogenicity of many chemical carcinogens and
their mutagenic activities [6,7]. Most tumor initiating agents either
generate or are metabolically converted to electrophilic reactants,
which bind covalently to cellular DNA and other macromolecules [8].
The Millers have proposed a general theory to explain the initial
event in chemical carcinogenesis. All chemical carcinogens that are
not electrophilic reactants must be converted into a chemically reactive electrophilic form which then reacts with some critical macro-
molecule to initiate the carcinogenic process [8]. Previous studies
have demonstrated a correlation between the skin carcinogenicity of
several polycyclic aromatic hydrocarbons (PAHs) and their ability to
bind covalently to DNA [9,10].

TABLE 2

Two-Stage Carcinogenesis Systems[a]

Organ System	Initiators	Promoters
Mouse skin	Polycyclic aromatic hydrocarbons (PAH), urethane, direct-acting electrophiles (epoxides, β-propiolactone, Bis chloromethylether, N-acetoxyacetylaminofluorene and N-methyl-N'-nitro-N-nitrosoguanidine (MNNG), nitrosamines, naphthylamines	Croton oil, phorbol esters, fatty acids and fatty acid esters, surface-active agents, linear long chain alkanes, tobacco smoke condensate and extracts of unburned tobacco, certain euphorbia macrocyclic diterpenes, citrus oil, anthraline and other phenols
Rat & mouse liver	2-acetamidofluorene diethylnitrosamine, 2-methyl-N,N'-dimethyl-4-aminoazobenzene	Phenobarbital, DDT; Butylated hydroxytoluene, (BHT); polychlorobiphenyls, (PCB)
Mouse lung	Urethan, PAH	BHT, phorbol
Rat colon	Dimethylhydrazine	Bile acids, high fat diet, high cholesterol diet
Rat bladder	N-methyl-N-nitrosourea	Saccharin, cyclamate

Rat & mouse mammary gland	PAH	Hormones, high fat diet, phorbol
Rat stomach	MNNG	Surfactants
Rat esophagus	Diethylnitrosamine	Diet
Mouse cell culture systems	PAH, radiation	Phorbol esters, saccharin
Rat tracheal cell culture system	MNNG, PAH	Phorbol esters

[a]See [5] for details.

Tumor Promotion

In addition to causing inflammation and epidermal hyperplasia, the
phorbol ester tumor promoters have been shown to have several other
morphological and biochemical effects on the skin. These responses
to phorbol ester tumor promoters are summarized in Table 3. Of all
the observed phorbol ester related effects on the skin, the induction

TABLE 3
Morphological and Biochemical Responses of Mouse Skin
to Phorbol Ester Tumor Promoters

Responses	References
Induction of imflammation and hyperplasia	1,37
Induction of dark cells	12-14
Induction of morphological changes in adult skin resembling papillomas and carcinoma cells	12-14
An initial increase in keratinization followed by a decrease	12
Increase in DNA, RNA and protein synthesis	51
Increase in phospholipid synthesis	52
Increase in histone synthesis and phosphorylation	53,54
Increase in ornithine decarboxylase activity followed by increase in polyamines	15
Decrease in histidase activity	55
Induction of embryonic proteins in adult skin	56
Increase in protease activity	45
Decrease in the isoproterenol stimulation of cAMP	57
Decrease response of G_1 chalone in adult skin	58
Increase in protein kinase activity[a]	
Increase in prostaglandin synthesis	59,60

[a]M. Mamrack, S. M. Fischer, and T. J. Slaga (manuscript in preparation).

of epidermal cell proliferation, ornithine decarboxylase (ODC) and dark basal keratinocytes correlate best [11-15].

It is difficult to determine which of the many phorbol ester tumor promoter related responses are essential components of the promotion process. There is a good correlation between the promoting abilities of a series of phorbol esters and their ability to stimulate epidermal hyperplasia [11]; however, the correlation fails if one looks at nonphorbol ester hyperplastic agents[16]. O'Brien et al. [15] have reported an excellent correlation between the tumor promoting ability of various compounds (phorbol esters as well as nonphorbol ester compounds) and their ability to induce ODC activity in mouse skin. However, the diterpene mezerein, similar to TPA but with weak promoting activity, was found to induce ODC comparable to that of TPA [17].

Raick [18], using the electron microscope, found that phorbol ester tumor promoters induced the appearance of "dark basal cells" in the epidermis. An epidermal hyperplastic agent with very weak promoting activity, ethylphenylpropiolate (EPP), did not induce dark cells [18]. In addition, wounding induced a few dark cells which correlated with its ability as a weak promoter [13,14,17]. Furthermore, a large number of these dark cells are found in embryonic skin [14] and papillomas and carcinomas [13,14]. Slaga et al. [19] has reported that TPA induced 3 to 5 times the number of dark cells as mezerein. This ability to induce a phenotype similar to primitive stem cells was the first major difference found between these compounds (Table 4).

TABLE 4
Induction of Dark Cells in Epidermis Following Several Treatments

Treatment	Characteristics	Dark Cell Induction
DMBA	Subcarcinogenic dose	-
TPA	Strong promoter	++++
Mezerein	Weak promoter	+
EPP	Very weak promoter	+/-
Wounding	Weak promoter	+

Epidermal Protein Kinases

Recent work in our laboratory has attempted to correlate changes in
protein phosphorylation with the tumor promotion process. We have
found that TPA causes a 2-3 fold increase in a cAMP independent protein
kinase activity [E. C. 2.7.1.37] 24 to 72 hours after a single application of 2-4 mg (Table 5). This enzyme activity has been partially
purified and been shown to phosphorylate a specialized epidermal structural protein in vitro. In addition, this kinase activity has the
capacity to phosphorylate tyrosine residues as well as serine and
threonine.

The enzymes which catalyze the post-translational phosphorylation
of proteins have generally been classified as either cyclic nucleotide
regulated or cyclic nucleotide independent [20]. The cyclic nucleotide
protein kinases are not under direct control of either cAMP or cGMP
or the same regulatory proteins as the cyclic nucleotide regulated
enzymes. Cyclic nucleotide independent protein kinases have been
partially purified from a variety of tissues with highly purified enzyme preparations reported from yeast [21], Novikoff ascites tumor
cells [22], human erythrocytes [23], and rabbit reticulocytes [24].

The cyclic nucleotide independent kinases have a number of other
properties which distinguish them from the cyclic nucleotide regulated
kinases. The independent kinases in general prefer acidic proteins
such as phosvitin or casein as substrates in contrast to basic proteins
such as histones which are phosphate acceptors for the cyclic nucleotide regulated enzymes. The independent enzymes are often referred
to as "casein", "phosvitin" or "phosphoprotein" kinases. At least
two different types of these activities have been reported [24,25].
They differ in some other properties which distinguish this class of
enzymes. These include the ability to substitute GTP for ATP, stimulation by monovalent salts, and the ability to bind phosphocellulose
in addition to DEAE cellulose [21-26]. However, the physiological
function and the in vivo substrates for this class of enzymes is
unknown.

TABLE 5
Relative Kinase Activity[a]

	24 hr	48 hr	72 hr
Control	100	100	100
EPP (14 mg)	117	130	185
Mezerein (2 ug)	183	147	160
TPA (2 ug)	117	185	205

[a]Extracts (10 mM NaCl, 10 mM Tris, pH 7.5,
1.5 mM $MgCl_2$) from treated animals (5 per
group) were separated on phosphocellulose columns by stepwise elution. Activity eluting
with 1.1 M NaCl is presented. The [^{32}P] radioactivity transferred to TCA precipitable casein
in 30 min per ug DNA is expressed relative to
acetone treated control animals.

Male Sencar mice, 6-8 weeks old, were treated with TPA and after
a period of time the epidermis was separated from the dermis and extracted with a hypotonic buffer (10 mM NaCl, 1.5 mM $MgCl_2$, 10 mM Tris,
pH 7.5). The extract was first chromatographed on DEAE cellulose;
the major peak of activity eluting at 0.3 M to 0.4 M NaCl was separated
further on a phosphocellulose column. The characterization of the
peak of activity eluting at about 0.8 M NaCl is presented in Figure 1.
Figure 1A shows that the kinase reaction is linear for at least 60
minutes with either casein or stratum corneum basic protein (SCBP)
as the protein substrate. SCBP, generously donated by Dr. Beverly
Dale (Seattle, WA), is a specialized structural protein of the epidermis responsible for aggregating keratin fibrils into macrofilaments
[27,28]. The inactive precursor form is a phosphoprotein localized
in keratin-hyalin granules. The purified SCBP can act as an efficient
substrate for this enzyme activity in vitro. One of the distinguishing
traits of this enzyme activity is the apparent stimulation by monovalent cations. This is presented in Figure 1B. Figure 1C demonstrates two other properties of the enzyme activity: 1) stimulation

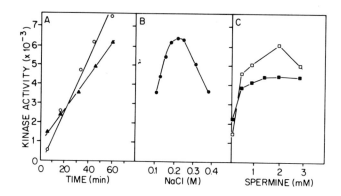

Figure 1. Characterization of protein kinase activity. Protein kinase G1 was partially purified by DEAE-cellulose and phosphocellulose chromatography. A. Time course of incorporation of ^{32}P into casein (o——o) or SCBP (▲——▲) from ATP by partially purified protein kinase G1. Incubation was at 37° for time indicated. B. Stimulation of kinase by NaCl with casein and ATP as substrates and kinase G1 incubated at 37° for 30 min. C. Stimulation of kinase activity G1 by spermine with either ATP (□——□) or GTP (■——■) as phosphate donor. Incubation conditions same as B with final concentration of NaCl at 0.2 M.

by polyamines with substitution of spermidine for spermine giving comparable results and 2) GTP can substitute for ATP as the phosphate donor. The difference in the level of stimulation is probably not due to the triphosphate donor, but rather to the age of the preparation as the polyamine effect decays with storage time at 4°.

No effect was observed on enzyme activity with the addition of cyclic AMP or cyclic GMP at concentrations ranging from 10^{-3} M to 10^{-7} M. In addition, the heat stable inhibitor protein [29] also had no effect. Therefore, this kinase activity can be classified as a cAMP independent kinase [30], sharing many of the properties of the Type III kinase described by Traugh and Traut [26].

It was of interest to determine the effect of various tumor promoters on the level of this enzyme activity. Table 6 presents some of the preliminary data. TPA causes the greatest increase in kinase activity per ug DNA relative to vehicle (acetone) treated control animals. EPP and mezerein also stimulated the kinase activity, but to a lesser extent with the EPP stimulation occurring 24-48 hours later than TPA.

TABLE 6

Quantitation of Phosphotyrosine in Epidermal Extracts Labeled In Vitro

| Treatment | Experiment 1[a] | | | Experiment 2[b] | |
	$\dfrac{\text{CPM Tyr (P)}}{\text{ug DNA}}$	% Tyr (P)[c]		$\dfrac{\text{CPM Tyr (P)}}{\text{ug protein}}$	$\dfrac{\text{CPM Tyr (P)}}{\text{ug DNA}}$
Control	34.5	12.2		3.8	20.2
EPP	59.6	14.3		3.2	29.8
MEZ	54.7	10.8		3.4	32.9
TPA	62.3	15.9		6.3	58.0

[a]Exp. 1: 48 hr time point with ATP as phosphate donor.
[b]Expt. 2: 72 hr time point with GTP as phosphate donor.
[c]% Tyr (P) = [Tyr (P)/Tyr (P) + Thr (P)] X 100.

Recent reports have shown increased phosphorylation of tyrosine residues in proteins from cells transformed by Rous sarcoma virus [30]. In addition, the transforming gene product of the virus has cAMP independent protein kinase activity (pp60^{src}) specific for tyrosine [31]. Uninfected cells also have a similar protein kinase (pp60^{sarc}) but present at 1/50 the level of infected cells [30,31]. Since TPA can also reversibly induce a transformed phenotype [5,31-35] and stimulate a protein kinase activity that shares some properties with the src gene product, the nature of the phosphorylated amino acids was examined.

Initial experiments showed a two-fold increase in phosphotyrosine (cpm/ug DNA) after TPA treatment. Three criteria were used to identify the radioactive spot as phosphotyrosine. First, the mobility relative to inorganic phosphate was virtually identical to that reported by others [30,31]. Second, the radioactivity eluted from the spot was resistant to treatment with 1M KOH at 55° for 2 hr, conditions which hydrolyze serine and threonine phosphate esters in peptides [36]. Thirdly, fluorescence analysis of the elutants revealed a pattern very similar to standard tyrosine with maximum excitation at about 280 nm.

The analysis of Tyr(P) was repeated with extracts from animals treated 72 hours previously with EPP, mezerein, and TPA. Radioactive GTP was the phosphate donor. Quantitation is given in Table 6. The greatest apparent stimulation is when the numbers are based on DNA. When Tyr(P) is expressed as a percentage of total phosphorylated amino acids, the values are similar which probably reflects the selective labeling conditions and suggests a quantitative effect as opposed to an altered enzyme form after a single TPA treatment.

Recently, Collet et al. [31] have shown that pp60^{src} can phosphorylate tyrosine residues specifically in a variety of structural proteins in vitro, including actin, desmin, 10 uM filaments and microtubules. This was of interest because cells transformed with temperature sensitive mutants of pp60^{src} rapidly revert to a more normal morphology after shifting to the nonpermissive temperature. The correlation between cell transformation and increased tyrosine phosphorylation has also been made by Hunter and Sefton [30]. The finding

that TPA causes an increase in a protein kinase activity that can
phosphorylate tyrosine raises intriguing questions concerning the mechanism of action of TPA. TPA has also been reported to partially mimic
viral infection in chick embryo fibroblasts [32-34] as well as produce
a transformed phenotype at the nonpermissive temperature in cells infected with temperature-sensitive mutants of Rous sarcoma virus [35].
The relationship between $pp60^{sarc}$ and other known cellular protein
kinases is unclear at this point. The role of tyrosine phosphorylation
in cell transformation and whether TPA can induce host cell $pp60^{sarc}$
expression are areas currently being investigated.

Multistage Promotion

It has recently been reported that mezerein is capable of bringing
about most of the morphological and biochemical changes in skin and
in cells in culture that TPA does, but TPA is at least 50 times more
active as a tumor promoter [17]. A comparison of these TPA and mezerein responses are shown in Table 7. Mezerein is as potent or more
potent than TPA in the induction of epidermal ODC and epidermal hyperplasia. The effect of mezerein on ODC activity suggests that ODC induction is not a critical event in tumor promotion [17]. It should
be emphasized that this is also true for the other morphological and
biochemical responses to mezerein.

Because of the many similarities in morphological and biochemical
responses induced by TPA and mezerein, it was felt that mezerein, although a weak promoter, could be effective in the second stage of a
two-stage promotion protocol as originally reported by Boutwell [37].
This lab recently reported that mezerein was indeed a potent stage II
promoter [19,38]. Boutwell showed that promotion could be divided
into two steps, conversion and propagation [37]. After DMBA initiation, the conversion stage was accomplished by a limited number of
croton oil treatments which, with no further treatment, only produced
a few tumors. The propagation stage was accomplished by repeated
treatment with turpentine, a non-promoting hyperplastic agent [37].

TABLE 7
Comparison of Cellular and Biochemical Responses to TPA and Mezerein

	Relative Response[a]		Reference
	TPA	Mezerein	
Enhancement of neoplastic pheno-type	100	100	61
Promotion of neoplastic transfor-mation (C3H-10T 1/2)	100	80	62,63[b]
Induction of epidermal cellular proliferation	50	100	1,17
Co-mitogenesis in lymphocytes	100	100	64
Inhibition of differentiation in FL cells	100	100	61,65
Stimulation of DNA synthesis	50	100	17[c]
Stimulation of ODC activity	80	100	17[c]
Stimulation of plasminogen activator production	20	100	61

[a]For a comparative purpose the maximum response of mezerein or TPA is expressed as a 100. The values should only be considered as an approximation.
[b]Personal communication from S. Mondal and C. Heidelberger.
[c]Manuscript in preparation by C. E. Weeks, S. M. Fischer and T. J. Slaga.

The three-stage protocol (initiation-conversion-propagation) produced a significant tumor response but less than that observed when croton oil was given for the complete promotion stage [37]. However, although the above experiments were repeatable at that time, more recent results showed that very weakly promoting hyperplastic agents, given repetitively after a few treatments of TPA, were not able to complete the promotion process as reported by Boutwell [13,16,18]. In fact, Raick reported that turpentine and EPP gave fewer tumors in a three-stage system than when DMBA was followed only by limited TPA treatment [13, 18]. Similar results were reported by Slaga et al. [16] using acetic

TABLE 8

Two-Stage Tumor Promotion After DMBA Initiation[a]

Exp. No.	Treatment Protocol — 21 weeks —	Tumor Response pap/mouse	% of Mice With Tumors
1 DMBA 1 wk →TPA 2X/wk for 20 wks		8.2	100
2 DMBA 1 wk →TPA 2X/wk for 2 wks acetone 2X/wk for 18 wks		0	0
3 DMBA 1 wk →mezerein 2 ug 2X/wk for 20 wks		0	0
4 DMBA 1 wk →mezerein 4 ug 2X/wk for 20 wks		0.2	18
5 DMBA 1 wk →TPA 2X/wk for 2 wks mezerein 1 ug 2X/wk for 18 wks		2.1	60
6 DMBA 1 wk →TPA 2X/wk for 2 wks mezerein 2 ug 2X/wk for 18 wks		4.0	90
7 DMBA 1 wk →TPA 2X/wk for 2 wks mezerein 4 ug 2X/wk for 18 wks		7.1	100
8 DMBA 1 wk →acetone 2X/wk for 2 wks mezerein 4 ug 2X/wk for 18 wks		0.1	10
9 DMBA 1 wk →EPP (14 mg) 2X/wk for 20 wks		0.1	10
10 DMBA 1 wk →TPA 2X/wk for 2 wks EPP (14 mg) 2X/wk for 18 wks		0.2	12

[a]The mice were initiated with 10 nmole of DMBA and followed one week later by twice weekly applications of 2 ug of TPA for 2 weeks. Starting on the third week of promotion the mice received either twice weekly applications of various dose levels of mezerein, EPP or only acetone. 95% or greater of the mice were alive at the end of the experimental period. The maximum percent standard deviation for the experiments was 16%.

acid as a second step promoter. It should be pointed out that turpentine, EPP and acetic acid do not induce many of the biochemical
responses induced by TPA and mezerein even though they are hyperplastic
agents. The variable response of turpentine as a stage II promoter
may be because it is a variable complex mixture.

A summary of the results on the use of mezerein as a second stage
promoter in two-stage promotion are shown in Table 8. As illustrated,
TPA is about 50 times more active as a promoter than mezerein (compare
experiments 1, 3 and 4). When 2 ug of TPA are given twice weekly for
only 2 weeks after DMBA initiation, no tumors are induced compared
to twice weekly treatments for 18 weeks. However, when mezerein is
given at a dose of either 1, 2, or 4 ug twice weekly after the limited
TPA treatment, it induced a significant tumor response in a dose-
dependent manner (compare experiments 5, 6, 7 with 2). The ability
of mezerein to act as a potent second stage promoter was repeated in
ten separate experiments [19,38]. Also shown in Table 8 is the in-
effectiveness of EPP as a complete promoter and as a second stage
promoter.

Inhibitors of Tumor Promotion

Various modifiers of the tumor promotion process have been very useful
in our understanding of the mechanisms of tumor promotion. Table 9
summarizes the potent inhibitors of skin tumor promotion in mice by
phorbol ester tumor promoters. The anti-inflammatory steroid fluo-
cinolone acetonide (FA), was found to be extremely potent inhibitor
of phorbol ester tumor promotion in mouse skin. FA also effectively
counteracts the tumor promoter induced cellular proliferation. Certain
retinoids are also potent inhibitors of mouse skin tumor promotion
[39-41]. In addition, Sporn and coworkers have found that certain
retinoids are potent inhibitors of lung, mammary, bladder and colon
carcinogenesis [42]. Verma and coworkers [39-41] have shown that certain retinoids are potent inhibitors of phorbol ester induced epidermal
ODC activity. We have recently found that a combination of FA and
retinoids produces an inhibitory effect on skin tumor promotion greater

TABLE 9
Inhibitors of Phorbol Ester Skin Tumor Promotion

Inhibitors	Reference
Anti-inflammatory steroids: cortisol, dexamethasone and fluocinolone acetonide	50
Vitamin A derivatives	39-41
Combination of retinoids and anti-inflammatory agents	
Protease inhibitors: Tosyl lysine chloromethyl ketone, (TLCK); Tosyl arginine methyl ester, (TAME); Tosyl phenylalanine chloromethyl ketone, (TPCK); antipain and leupeptin	43
Cyclic nucleotides	44,45
Dimethylsulfoxide (DMSO)	44
Butyrate	44
Bacillus Calmette-Guerin (BCG)	47
Polyriboinosinic:polyribocytidylic acid (Poly I:C)	48

than that produced by each separately [43]. Troll and Belmain [44-46] have found that protease inhibitors, cyclic nucleotides, DMSO and buty- rate also inhibit mouse skin tumor promotion by phorbol esters. Schinitsky and coworkers [47] reported the inhibitory effect of Bacillus Calmette-Guerin (BCG) vaccination on skin tumor promotion. It has been shown that Polyriboinosinic-polyribocytidylic (Poly I:C) has an inhibitory effect on carcinogenesis and tumor promotion [48]. This appears to be mediated by its inhibition of promoter and carcinogen induced cell proliferation [49].

The effectiveness of some of the inhibitors of tumor promotion on two-stage promotion was recently reported [49]. The effects of FA, retinoic acid, (RA), and tosyl phenylalanine chloromethyl ketone (TPCK) on two-stage promotion are shown in Table 10. As shown in Experiments 1 and 2 of Table 10, stages I and II of promotion separate- ly do not cause tumors to develop after DMBA initiation when given

TABLE 10

The Effects of RA, FA and TPCK on Two-Stage Promotion After DMBA Initiation[a]

Exp. No.	Treatment Protocol ←——— 21 weeks ———→	Tumor Response	
		No. of Papillomas Per Mouse	% of Mice w/Tumors
1	DMBA $\xrightarrow{1\ wk}$ TPA 2X/wk for 2 wks	0	0
2	DMBA $\xrightarrow{1\ wk}$ acetone 2X/wk for 2 wks $\xrightarrow{mezerein}$ 2X/wk for 18 wks	0	0
3	DMBA $\xrightarrow{1\ wk}$ TPA 2X/wk for 2 wks $\xrightarrow{mezerein}$ 2X/wk for 18 wks	4.2	92
4	DMBA $\xrightarrow{1\ wk}$ TPA + FA (1 ug) 2X/wk for 2 wks $\xrightarrow{mezerein}$ 2X/wk for 18 wks	0	0
5	DMBA $\xrightarrow{1\ wk}$ TPA + FA (0.1 ug) 2X/wk for 2 wks $\xrightarrow{mezerein}$ 2X/wk for 18 wks	0.4	26
6	DMBA $\xrightarrow{1\ wk}$ TPA 2X/wk for 2 wks $\xrightarrow{mezerein + FA\ (1\ ug)}$ 2X/wk for 18 wks	0.8	35
7	DMBA $\xrightarrow{1\ wk}$ TPA + RA (10 ug) 2X/wk for 2 wks $\xrightarrow{mezerein}$ 2X/wk for 18 wks	4.0	88
8	DMBA $\xrightarrow{1\ wk}$ TPA 2X/wk for 2 wks $\xrightarrow{mezerein + RA\ (10\ ug)}$ 2X/wk for 18 wks	0.8	34
9	DMBA $\xrightarrow{1\ wk}$ TPA + TPCK (10 ug) 2X/wk for 2 wks $\xrightarrow{mezerein}$ 2X/wk for 18 wks	1.0	40
10	DMBA $\xrightarrow{1\ wk}$ TPA 2X/wk for 2 wks $\xrightarrow{mezerein + TPCK\ (10\ ug)}$ 2X/wk for 18 wks	3.8	87

[a]The mice were initiated with 10 nmoles of DMBA and followed one week later by twice weekly applications of 2 ug of TPA for 2 weeks (stage I). Starting on the third week of promotion the mice received twice weekly applications of 2 ug of mezerein (stage 2). In some experiments FA, RA or TPCK were given simultaneously with either stage I or II. 98% or greater of the mice were alive at the end of the experimental period. The maximum percent standard deviation for the experiments was 14%.

under the treatment protocol shown. However, when stage I and II
agents are given sequentially after DMBA initiation, a significant
tumor response is seen (Experiment 3). FA is a potent inhibitor of
stages I and II of promotion but to a greater degree for stage I than
stage II. It should be emphasized that only 4 applications of FA
with TPA were necessary to counteract the tumor response. RA was
ineffective in stage I but was a potent inhibitor of stage II promotion. TPCK specifically inhibited stage I but not stage II. These
results were reported previously [19,38,49].

Since the only major morphological or biochemical difference between the effects of TPA and mezerein on the skin is the ability of
TPA to induce a large number of dark basal keratinocytes [13,14], we
investigated the effects of various inhibitors of promotion on the
appearance of dark cells. If dark cells are critical in the first
stage of promotion and if FA and TPCK are potent inhibitors of stage
I and RA of stage II, then only FA and TPCK should counteract the
appearance of these cells. As hypothesized, FA and TPCK were both
found to effectively counteract the appearance of the dark cells induced by TPA, whereas RA had no effect [49].

Since TPCK is a potent inhibitor of stage I of promotion but
not of stage II and since TPCK counteracted the TPA-induced increase
in the dark basal keratinocytes, the effect of TPCK on TPA-induced
ODC activity was analyzed. TPCK had very little effect on TPA- and
mezerein-induced epidermal ODC activity; this was even evident at a
relatively high TPCK dose level (20 ug) [49]. The anti-inflammatory
steroid FA not only counteracted the appearance of dark cells induced
by TPA, but also suppressed the hyperplasia induced by TPA. In fact,
the skins from FA plus TPA treated mice appeared morphologically as
untreated skin. This is in agreement with our previously reported
observations on the inhibitory effect of FA on TPA induced inflammation, hyperplasia and DNA synthesis [50]. TPCK appeared to have only
a slight inhibitory effect on TPA induced inflammation and hyperplasia
[49].

Although RA inhibited stage II or promotion, it had no inhibitory effect on the TPA or mezerein induced hyperplasia. However, certain retinoids are potent inhibitors of TPA and mezerein induced epidermal ODC activity [39-41]. These data suggest that the induction of epidermal ODC activity followed by increased polyamines may be important in stage II of promotion. In this regard, FA and TPCK have either no effect or only a slight inhibitory effect on TPA or mezerein induced ODC activity [43,49]. FA does, however, significantly decrease the TPA induced spermidine levels in the epidermis [43]. This decrease, plus FA's inhibitory effect on TPA induced hyperplasia, may be responsible for its inhibitory effect on stage II promotion.

SUMMARY

The data presented from this laboratory suggest that at least two stages are important in the promotion process, both of which can obviously be produced by repeated TPA treatment after tumor initiation. We believe that one of the important events in the first stage involves the induction of dark basal keratinocytes. Mezerein is a potent second stage promoter, but only a weak complete promoter with much less ability to induce dark cells than TPA. In addition, FA and TPCK inhibit stage I of promotion and inhibit the induction of dark cells by TPA whereas RA does not, suggesting that the dark cells are important in stage I of promotion (Figure 2). These dark basal keratinocytes are slightly increased by wounding which correlates with its relatively weak promoting ability but not by EPP, which is a very weak promoting hyperplastic agent [13,14,18,51]. In addition, a large number of these dark cells are found in papillomas and carcinomas [13,14]. These dark cells may be primitive stem cells since we have found (unpublished results), as have others [13,14], that they normally occur in large numbers in embryonic and newborn skin but are present in very small numbers in adult skin. It appears that the induction of ODC activity, followed by increased polyamines and increased cellular proliferation, are important events in stage II of

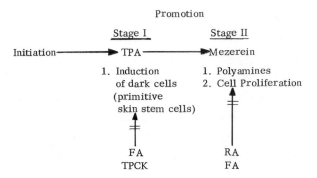

Figure 2. A diagram of the various stages of skin carcinogenesis showing the important events in stages I and II of promotion and where FA, RA and TPCK inhibit promotion.

promotion. The increase in a protein kinase activity by TPA with the capacity to phosphorylate tyrosine residues in epidermal proteins may be involved in the maintenance of a "transformed phenotype" similar to the Avian sarcoma virus coded protein kinase. Experiments are underway to more clearly define this event within the conversion-propagation model. Figure 2 depicts the various stages, the important events in each stage, and where the various inhibitors are effective. By seeking to divide the carcinogenic process operationally into as many stages as possible and finding specific inhibitors of each stage, we will have a greater opportunity to understand the carcinogenic process as well as providing a rational and effective basis for the prevention of cancer.

ABBREVIATIONS

BP, benzo(a)pyrene; DMBA, 7,12-dimethylbenzo(a)anthracene; TPA, 12-0-tetradecanoylphorbol-13-acetate; PAH, polycyclic aromatic hydrocarbons; ODC, ornithine decarboxylase; DMSO, dimethylsulfoxide; BCG, Bacillus Calmette-Guerin; EPP, ethylphenylpropiolate; TLCK, tosyl lysine chloromethyl ketone; TAME, tosyl arginine methyl ester; TPCK, tosyl phenylalanine chloromethyl ketone.

ACKNOWLEDGMENTS

This research was sponsored by U.S. EPA contract number 79-D-X0526
under Interagency Agreement DOE number 40-728-78 and the Office of
Health and Environmental Research, U.S. Department of Energy, under
contract W-7405-eng-26 with the Union Carbide Corporation.

Dr. Mamrack is a Postdoctoral Investigator supported by Training
Grant T32-CA09336 from the National Cancer Institute.

REFERENCES

1. Slaga, T. J., Scribner, J. D., Thompson, S., and Viaje, A., *J. Natl. Cancer Inst.*, *57*:1145-1159 (1976).

2. Slaga, T. J., Bowden, G. T., Scribner, J. D., and Boutwell, R. D., *J. Natl. Cancer Inst.*, *53*:1337-1340 (1974).

3. VanDuuren, B. L., *Progr. Exptl. Tumor Res.*, *11*:31-68 (1969).

4. VanDuuren, B. L., Sivak, A., Segal, A., Seidman, I., and Katz, C., *Cancer Res.*, *33*:2166-2172 (1973).

5. Slaga, T. J., Sivak, A., and Boutwell, R. K. (eds), Carcinogenesis: A Comprehensive Survey. Vol. 2, Mechanisms of Tumor Promotion and Cocarcinogenesis, Raven Press, N.Y., 1978.

6. McCann, J. and Amer, B. N., *Proc. Natl. Acad. Sci.*, *U.S.A.*, *73*: 950-954 (1976).

7. Huberman, E. J., *Environmental Pathology and Toxicology*, *2*:29-42 (1978).

8. Miller, E. C. and Miller, J. A., The metabolism of chemical carcinogens to reactive electrophiles and their possible mechanism of action in carcinogenesis. In: Chemical Carcinogens, C. E. Searle, Ed., ACS Washington, 1976, p. 732.

9. Brookes, P. and Lawley, P. D., *Nature*, *202*:781-784.

10. Slaga, T. J., Buty, S. G., Thompson, S., Bracken, W. M., and Viaje, A. A., *Cancer Res.*, *37*:3126-3131 (1977).

11. Slaga, T. J., Scribner, J. D., Thompson, S., and Viaje, A., *J. Natl. Cancer Inst.*, *52*:1611-1618 (1974).

12. Raick, A. N., *Cancer Res.*, *33*:269-286 (1973).

13. Raick, A. N., *Cancer Res.*, *34*:920-926 (1974).

14. Raick, A. N., *Cancer Res.*, *34*:2915-2925 (1974).

15. O'Brien, T. G., Simsiman, R. C., and Boutwell, R. K., *Cancer Res.*, *35*:1662-1670 (1975).

16. Slaga, T. J., Bowden, G. T., and Boutwell, R. K., *J. Natl. Cancer Inst.*, *55*:983-987 (1975).

17. Mufson, R. A., Fischer, S. M., Verma, A. K., Gleason, G. L., Slaga, T. J., and Boutwell, R. K., *Cancer Res.*, *39*:4791-4795 (1979).

18. Raick, A. N. and Burdzy, K., *Cancer Res.*, *33*:2221-2230 (1973).

19. Slaga, T. J., Fischer, S. M., Weeks, C. E., and Kelin-Szanto, A. J. P., Multistage chemical carcinogenesis. In: Biochemistry of Normal and Abnormal Epidermal Differentiation, (M. Seije and I. A. Bernstein, Eds.), Univ. of Tokyo Press, Tokyo (in press).

20. Rusin, C. S. and Rosen, O. M., *Ann. Rev. Biochem.*, *44*:831-887 (1975).

21. Lerch, K., Muir, L. W., and Fischer, E. E., *Biochem.*, *14*:2015-2023 (1975).

22. Dahmus, M. E. and Natzle, J., *Biochem.*, *16*:1901-1908 (1977).

23. Boivin, P. and Galand, C., *Biochem. Biophys. Res. Commun.*, *89*:7-16 (1979).

24. Hathaway, G. M. and Traugh, J. A., *J. Biol. Chem.*, *254*:762-768 (1979).

25. Cochet, C., Job, D., Pirollet, and Chambaz, E. M., *Endocrinol.*, *106*:750-757 (1980).

26. Traugh, S. A. and Traut, T. T., *J. Biol. Chem.*, *249*:1207-1212 (1974).

27. Dale, B. A. and Ling, S. U., *Biochem.*, *18*:3539-3546 (1979).

28. Lonsdale-Eccles, J. D., Haugen, J. A., and Dale, B. A., *J. Biol. Chem.*, *255*:2235-2238 (1980).

29. Walsh, D. A., Ashby, C. D., Genzalez, Calkins, D., Fischer, E. H., and Krebs, E. G., *J. Biol. Chem.*, *246*:1977-1985 (1971).

30. Hunter, T. and Sefton, B. M., *Proc. Natl. Acad. Sci., U.S.A.,*
     77:1311-1315 (1980).

31. Collett, M. S., Purchio, A. F., and Erikson, R. L., *Nature, 285:*
     167-169 (1980).

32. Driedger, P. E. and Blumberg, P. M., *Cancer Res., 37*:3257-3265
     (1977).

33. Weinstein, I. B., Wigler, M., and Pietropaolo, C., In: Origins
     of Human Cancer (H. H. Hiatt, J. D. Watson and J. A. Winsten,
     eds.), Cold Spring Harbor, New York, 1977, pp. 751-772.

34. Delclos, K. B. and Blumberg, P. M., *Cancer Res., 39*:1667-1672
     (1979).

35. Bissell, M. J., Hatre, C., and Calvin, M., *Proc. Natl. Acad.
     Sci., U.S.A., 76*:348-352 (1979).

36. Bitte, L. and Kabat, D., *Methods Enzymol., 30*:563-590 (1974).

37. Boutwell, R. K., *Progr. Exptl. Tumor Res., 4*:207-250 (1964).

38. Slaga, T. J., Fischer, S. M., Nelson, K., and Gleason, G. L.,
     Proc. Natl. Acad. Sci., U.S.A., 77:3659-3663 (1980).

39. Verma, A. K. and Boutwell, R. K., *Cancer Res., 37*:2196-2201
     (1977).

40. Verma, A. K., Rice, H. M., Shapas, B. G., and Boutwell, R. K.,
     Cancer Res., 38:793-801 (1978).

41. Verma, A. K., Shapas, B. G., Rice, H. M., and Boutwell, R. K.,
     Cancer Res., 39:419-424 (1979).

42. Sporn, M. B., Dunlop, N. M., and Newton, D. L., *Fed. Proc., 35:*
     1332-1337 (1976).

43. Weeks, C. E., Slaga, T. J., Hennings, H., Gleason, G. L., and
     Bracken, W. M., *J. Natl. Cancer Inst., 63*:401-406 (1979).

44. Belman, S. and Troll, W., Hormones, cyclic nucleotides and pros-
     taglandins. In: Carcinogenesis, Vol. 2 (T. J. Slaga, A. Sivak
     and R. K. Boutwell, eds.), Raven Press, New York, 1978, pp. 117-
     134.

45. Troll, W., Meyn, M. S., and Tossman, T. G., Mechanisms of pro-
     tease action in carcinogenesis. In: Carcinogenesis, Vol. 2
     (T. J. Slaga, A. Sivak and R. K. Boutwell, eds.), Raven Press,
     New York, 1978, pp. 301-312.

46. Belman, S. and Troll, W., *Cancer Res., 34*:3446-3451 (1974).

47. Schinitsky, M. R., Hyman, L. R., Blazkovec, A. A., and Burkholder, P. M., *Cancer Res., 33*:659-663 (1973).

48. Gelboin, H. V. and Levy, H. B., *Science, 167*:205-207 (1970).

49. Slaga, T. J., Klein-Szanto, A. J. P., Fischer, S. M., Weeks, C. E., Nelson, K., and Major, S., *Proc. Natl. Acad. Sci., U.S.A., 77*:2251-2254 (1980).

50. Slaga, T. J., Fischer, S. M., Viaje, A., Berry, D. L., Bracken, W. M., LeClerc, S., and Miller, D. L., Inhibition of tumor promotion by anti-inflammatory agents: An approach to the biochemical mechanism of promotion. In: Carcinogenesis, Vol. 2 (T. J. Slaga, A. Sivak and R. K. Boutwell, eds.), Raven Press, N.Y. (1978) pp. 173-195.

51. Baird, W. M., Sedgwick, J. A., and Boutwell, R. K., *Cancer Res., 31*:1434-1439 (1971).

52. Rohrschneider, L. R., O'Brien, D. H., and Boutwell, R. K., *Biochim. Biophys. Acta., 280*:57-70 (1972).

53. Raineri, R., Simsiman, R. C., and Boutwell, R. K., *Cancer Res., 33*:134-139 (1973).

54. Raineri, R., Simsiman, R. C., and Boutwell, R. K., *Cancer Res., 37*:4584-4589 (1977).

55. Colburn, W. H., Lau, S., and Head, R., *Cancer Res., 35*:3154-3159 (1975).

56. Balmain, A. J., *Invest. Dermatol., 67*:246-253 (1976).

57. Mufson, R. A., Simsiman, R. C., and Boutwell, R. K., *Cancer Res., 37*:665-669 (1977).

58. Krieg, L., Kuhlmann and Marks, F., *Cancer Res., 34*:3135-3146 (1974).

59. Verma, A. K., Ashendel, C. L., and Boutwell, R. K., *Cancer Res., 40*:308-315 (1980).

60. Bresnick, E., Meumer, P., and Lamden, M., *Cancer Letters, 7*:121-125 (1979).

61. Weinstein, I. B., Wigler, M., and Pietropaolo, C., The action of tumor promoting agents in cell culture. In: (H. H. Heatt, J. D. Watson and J. A. Winsten, eds.), Cold Spring Harbor Laboratory (1977), pp. 751-772.

62. Heidelberger, C., Mondal, S. and Peterson, A. R., Initiation
     and promotion in cell cultures. In: Carcinogenesis, Vol. 2
     (T. J. Slaga, A. Sivak and R. K. Boutwell, eds.), Raven Press,
     New York, pp. 197-202.

63. Mondal, S. and Heidelberger, C., *Nature, 260:*710-711 (1976).

64. Kensler, T. W. and Mueller, G. C., *Cancer Res., 38:*771-775.

65. Diamond, L., O'Brien, T. and Rovera, G., Tumor promoters inhibit
     terminal cell differentiation in culture. In: Carcinogenesis,
     Vol. 2 (T. J. Slaga, A. Sivak and R. K. Boutwell, eds.), Raven
     Press, New York (1978), pp. 335-341.

THE EFFECT OF TUMOR-CAUSING CHEMICALS ON THE CONTROL OF MUTAGENESIS AND DIFFERENTIATION IN MAMMALIAN CELLS

Carol A. Jones
Eliezer Huberman

Toxicology and Carcinogenesis Program
Biology Division
Oak Ridge National Laboratory
Oak Ridge, Tennessee

SUMMARY

A cell-mediated mutagenesis assay was developed to study the potential carcinogenic hazard of some environmental chemicals. In this assay, Chinese hamster V79 cells, which are susceptible to mutagenesis, are co-cultivated with cells capable of metabolizing chemical carcinogens. This assay made it possible to demonstrate a relationship between the degrees of carcinogenicity and mutagenicity of a series of polycyclic hydrocarbons and nitrosamines and to study the organ specificity exhibited by some chemical carcinogens. However, most short-term in vitro assays are designed to detect mutagenic activity and therefore do not detect tumor-promoting agents that are devoid of this activity. By analyzing various markers of terminal differentiation in cultured human melanoma and myeloid leukemia cells, we have established a relationship between the activity of a series of tumor-promoting phorbol diesters in mouse skin and their ability to induce terminal differentiation. We suggest that measuring alterations in the differentiation characteristics of some cultured cells may represent an approach by which environmental tumor-promoting agents can be studied and detected.

INTRODUCTION

Many industrial chemicals introduced each year into our environment
[1] may be responsible for a significant proportion of human cancers
[2]. While the mechanism by which chemicals induce cancer is not
known, one major concept is the somatic mutation theory, which suggests
that malignancy results from the alterations produced by carcinogens
in the genetic material of exposed cells. Studies demonstrating the
capacity of carcinogens to bind to the DNA of susceptible mammalian
cells [3-8] and to induce mutations [9-10] support this hypothesis.
It is presumed that such mutations involve the genes controlling the
expression of malignant transformation [11-14]. Therefore, studying
the mutagenic activity of carcinogens in mammalian cells could be useful in elucidating the genetic events most likely to result in malignant transformation and could provide an important technique for the
identification of potential carcinogens [15-21]. Most chemicals are
not carcinogenic per se but require metabolic activation before they
can manifest their biological activity [22-23]. However, mammalian
cells used as the target cells for inducing genetic damage are usually
unable to metabolize carcinogens [24-27]. To overcome this limitation,
an exogenous metabolic activation system is added. The activation
systems most commonly used are liver microsomal or S9 preparations
[19,28-30], which will not necessarily metabolize compounds in a manner
analogous to that of intact cells [18,31,32]. We have therefore introduced into the mutagenesis studies intact cells for the carcinogen
metabolism; we call this approach the cell-mediated mutagenesis assay
[17,18,32-35].

Cell-Mediated Mutagenesis

In the cell-mediated assay, we cultivate Chinese hamster V79 cells,
which are useful for mutagenesis [15] but are unable to activate carcinogens [17,27,33], with lethally irradiated fibroblasts [17,27] or
primary hepatocytes [33,35], which can metabolize chemical carcinogens.
The reactive intermediates produced by the metabolizing cells are

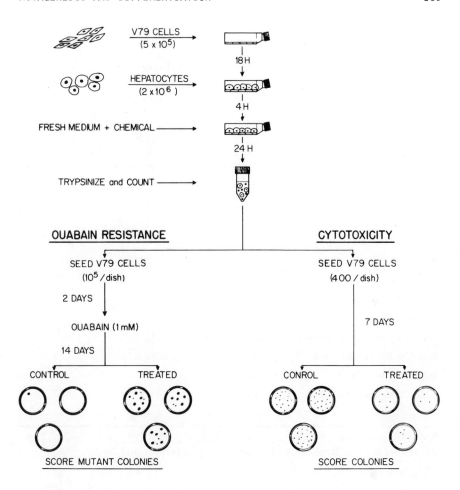

Figure 1. Scheme for the induction of ouabain-resistant mutants in the hepatocyte-mediated assay (reprinted with permission from Jones and Huberman [31]).

apparently transferred to the V79 cells, where they induce mutations. After exposure to the carcinogen the cultures are dissociated, and the V79 cells are subcultured for the determination of cell survival and, under appropriate conditions, for the determination of mutation frequencies at genetic markers such as 8-azaguanine, 6-thioguanine, or ouabain resistance [15-19,22-30] (Figure 1).

TABLE 1
Induction of Ouabain-Resistant Mutants in the Fibroblast-Mediated
Assay by Carcinogenic Polycyclic Hydrocarbons After Treatment
With or Without Aminophylline[a]

Hydrocarbon	Concentration (μg/ml)	No. of Ouabain-Resistant Mutants Per 10^6 Survivors	
		Without Aminophylline	With Aminophylline
Control	0	1	1
Phenanthrene	1	1	1
Pyrene	1	1	1
Benzo(e)pyrene	1	1	NT[b]
Benz(a)anthracene	1	2	NT[b]
Chrysene	1	2	NT[b]
Dibenz(a,c)anthracene	1	3	5
Dibenz(a,h)anthracene	1	4	46
7-Methylbenz(a)anthracene	1	24	NT[b]
3-Methylcholanthrene	1	108	413
Benzo(a)pyrene	1	121	214
7,12-Dimethylbenz(a)-anthracene	0.1	66	NT[b]

[a]Cells were treated with 0.1 mM aminophylline. The data are based on results from Huberman [10] and from Huberman and Sachs [34].
[b]NT, not tested.

In the cell-mediated assay, using hamster embryonic fibroblasts as the metabolizing cells, we have established a relationship between the degree of mutagenicity and the degree of carcinogenicity for a series of polycyclic hydrocarbons [17,34] (Table 1). After co-cultivation, four carcinogenic aromatic hydrocarbons--such as 7,12-dimethyl-benz(a)anthracene, benzo(a)pyrene, 3-methylcholanthrene, and 7-methyl-benz(a)anthracene--induced drug-resistant mutants, whereas five non-carcinogenic hydrocarbons--such as benzo(e)pyrene, benz(a)anthracene, phenanthrene, pyrene, and chrysene--were inactive. The mutagenic activities of the carcinogenic hydrocarbons were dependent on the

number of metabolizing cells present and on the concentration of the
carcinogens. Dibenzo(a,c)anthracene and dibenzo(a,h)anthracene, which
have been reported to be non-carcinogenic in golden hamsters, showed
a weak mutagenic effect. In the presence of aminophylline, which enhances polycyclic aromatic hydrocarbon metabolism in the hamster embryo
cells [36], there was a two- to four-fold increase in mutagenicity
with benzo(a)pyrene and 3-methylcholanthrene (Table 1). Dibenzo(a,c)-
anthracene, which had a low degree of mutagenicity without aminophylline, showed less than a two-fold increase in mutagenicity with aminophylline. Dibenz(a,h)anthracene, which is a carcinogen for the mouse
and rat and which exhibited mutagenic activities similar to that of
dibenz(a,c)anthracene without aminophylline, showed a ten-fold increase
in mutagenicity with aminophylline (Table 1). These results indicate
a relationship between the degree of mutagenesis in the cell-mediated
system and the degree of carcinogenicity of polycyclic aromatic hydrocarbons.

In addition, by studying the mutagenic response of various metabolites and derivatives of a series of polycyclic aromatic hydrocarbons--
such as benz(a)anthracene [37], benzo(a)pyrene [38,39], and 7,12-
dimethylbenz(a)anthracene [40,49]--in the V79 cells co-cultivated with
or without fibroblasts, we have identified the metabolic pathway that
leads to the production of the diol epoxides [37-39] that are presumably the ultimate mutagenic forms of these carcinogens. Other studies
indicate that these metabolites are also the ones presumably responsible for induction of tumors in experimental animals.

The use of fibroblasts as metabolizing cells is limited since
they can metabolize only certain classes of carcinogens. Whereas
polycyclic hydrocarbons are efficiently activated by fibroblasts, many
classes of chemicals, including liver carcinogens, are not [42,43].
To further expand the use of the cell-mediated mutagenesis system,
we developed a system using primary rat hepatocytes to activate the
carcinogens and V79 cells to detect mutagenic metabolites [33,35]
(Figure 1). Hepatocytes were obtained after enzymic digestion of
perfused [44] or finely sliced [33,45] livers from adult rats. It
was found that hepatocytes prepared by the slicing method could

activate liver carcinogens such as nitrosamines more efficiently than
could hepatocytes prepared by the perfusion technique. In this im-
proved hepatocyte-mediated assay, the mutagenicity of nitrosamines
could be detected at dose levels that were 2-to-3 orders of magnitude
lower than those observed in other common short-term assays [33,46].
Furthermore, as in the case of the polycyclic hydrocarbons, we could
establish a relationship between the degree of mutagenicity of the
nitrosamines and the degree of carcinogenicity (Figure 2) [47]. In
view of this relationship and their ability to detect low levels of
carcinogens, these cell-mediated mutagenesis assays may, in addition

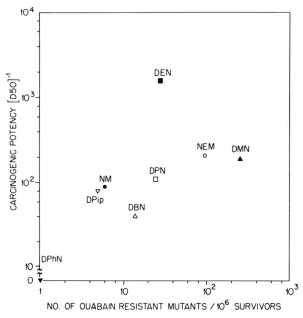

Figure 2. Relationship between the mutagenic activity of a series
of 8 nitrosamines and their carcinogenic potency. Mutagenic activi-
ty was defined by the number of ouabain-resistant mutants obtained
for 10^6 survivors following treatment with 100 µM of a nitrosamine.
Carcinogenic potencies were calculated according to the method of
Bartsch et al. [46] using the carcinogenesis data of rats from
Druckery et al. [47]. Abbreviations: DMN, N-nitrosodimethylamine;
NPip, 1-nitrosopiperidine; DBN, N-nitrosodibutylamine; DPN, N-nitro-
sodipropylamine; DPhN, N-nitrosodiphenylamine; NM, N-nitrosomorpholine;
NEM, N-nitrosoethylmethylamine; DEN, N-nitrosodiethylamine. (reprinted
with permission from Jones and Huberman [33]).

to their usefulness in mechanistic studies, serve as valuable tools
for screening chemicals hazardous to man.

Cell-Specificity in the Activation of Chemical Carcinogens into Mutagens

Many chemical carcinogens exhibit marked organ specificity in vivo,
but the critical factors that determine the susceptibility of an organ
to a given carcinogen remain largely unknown. The cell-mediated mutagenesis assay, which can use intact cells from various organs to metabolically activate chemical carcinogens, can be used as a means of
investigating the tissue specificity or cell specificity of chemical
carcinogens. To investigate such a cell specificity we compared the
abilities of rat fibroblasts (fibroblast-mediated assay) and hepatocytes (hepatocyte-mediated assay) (Figure 1) to activate several organ-
specific carcinogens. N-nitrosodimethylamine, which can produce liver
tumors but no fibrosarcomas, was activated into a potent mutagen by
hepatocytes but not by fibroblasts (Table 2). This lack of mutagenicity in the fibroblast-mediated assay may be explained by the absence
in the fibroblasts of the requisite metabolizing capacity for this
compound.

TABLE 2
Fibroblast- and Hepatocyte-Mediated Mutagenesis of V79 Cells
by the Carcinogens N-nitrosodimethylamine, Benzo(a)pyrene,
and 7,12-dimethylbenz(a)anthracene[a]

Metabolizing	No. of Ouabain-Resistant Mutants Per 10^6 Surviving V79 Cells		
	N-nitroso-dimethylamine	Benzo(a)pyrene	7,12-Dimethyl-benz(a)anthracene
None	1	1	1
Fibroblast	1	38	54
Hepatocyte	258	1	24

[a]The concentrations used were: 0.7 µg/ml N-nitrosodimethylamine and
1 µg/ml each of benzo(a)pyrene and 7,12-dimethylbenz(a)anthracene.

TABLE 3
Binding of Benzo(a)pyrene to Hepatocyte and Fibroblast DNA[a]

Concentration Benzo(a)pyrene (g/ml)	Hepatocytes (Benzo(a)pyrene residues/10^6 nucleosides)	Fibroblasts
0.01	0.67	0.26
0.1	10.0	1.47
1.0	31.5	3.34
12.0	147.0	ND[b]

[a]Primary liver cells (10×10^6) or fibroblasts (10×10^6) were treated
with benzo(a)pyrene or its metabolites for 18 h. The cell monolayer
was washed with phosphate-buffered saline and the cells dissociated
with trypsin. After extraction of the ce-lular DNA, the bound adducts
were separated by Sephadex LH-20 chromatography.
[b]ND - not determined.

Benzo(a)pyrene, a potent lung and skin carcinogen that can induce
fibrosarcomas but not liver tumors [48], was activated to a mutagen
for V79 cells by fibroblasts, but not by hepatocytes (Table 2). Unlike the case of N-nitrosodimethylamine, both hepatocytes and fibroblasts could extensively metabolize benzo(a)pyrene to products that
bind to the cellular DNA (Table 3) [49]. However, in the fibroblasts
the major benzo(a)pyrene adduct was derived from the reaction of diol
epoxide with the deoxyguanosine nucleosides (Figure 3). This adduct
is associated with the carcinogenic and mutagenic effects of benzo(a)-
pyrene [38,39,50]). By contrast, no diol epoxide adducts of benzo(a)-
pyrene were detected in the hepatocytes. In these cells, the major
adducts were hydrophilic nucleoside derivatives, which are presumably
non-mutagenic. In the hepatocyte- and fibroblast-mediated assays,
7,12-dimethylbenz(a)anthracene, which induces both liver tumors and
fibrosarcomas, was mutagenic (Table 2).

    In conclusion, our mutagenesis studies with mammalian cells pre-
sent a system that may (1) be predictive of carcinogenic potential,

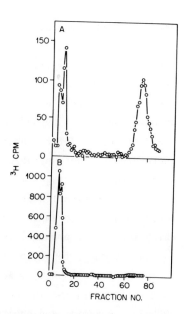

Figure 3. Binding of benzo(a)pyrene to hepatocyte and fibroblast DNA. Hepatocytes (10 X 10^6) or fibroblasts (10 X 10^6) were incubated with [^{3}H]-benzo(a)pyrene (1 µg/ml) for 18 h. After extraction of the cel- lular DNA, the bound adducts were separated by Sephadex LH-20 chroma- tography. The column was eluted with water until fraction 40, when the solvent was changed to methanol. (a) fibroblast DNA; (b) hepato- cyte DNA.

(2) be indicative of the organ specificity of a carcinogen, and (3) indicate the magnitude of the potential threat posed by a particular chemical.

Induction of Cell Differentiation by Tumor-Promoting Phorbol Diesters

The concept of carcinogenesis is one of a multi-stage process that is probably initiated by a mutation caused by the carcinogen and followed by a stepwise development resulting in the formation of tumors [51-53]. Studies have indicated that certain environmental agents may act by a non-mutagenic mechanism during the subsequent stages of the carcino- genesis process to promote tumor formation [51-54]. The action of these agents could be the rate-limiting determinants in human cancers. In view of this, it is important to elucidate both the mode of action

and the identity of environmental chemicals that may act as tumor
promoters. At the present time, the in vivo tests that can be used
to study and identify such chemicals are time consuming and require
large numbers of experimental animals. It is therefore important to
develop simple short-term in vitro cell assays. However, many of the
short-term assays, including bacterial [9,55] and mammalian cell systems [17,33,34,49], are designed to detect carcinogens by their mutagenic activity and, therefore, are not suitable for studying promoting
agents, many of which are devoid of mutagenic activity. Tumor promoters act most likely via a non-mutational event, presumably by altering
differentiation processes [51]. For example, phorbol-12-myristate-13-
acetate (PMA) [52], which is a tumor promoter in a two-stage carcinogenesis system [51-53], was recently found to alter cell differentiation in some avian and murine cells [56-61]. We have shown that PMA
can also induce terminal differentiation in some human cells, including
the promyelocytic HL60 [62], leukemia, and hamster ovary (HO) melanoma
cells [63]. Differentiation by PMA in the promyelocytic leukemia cells
could be induced at doses as low as 10^{-10} M. In the leukemia cells,
differentiation was determined by inhibition of cell growth, increase
in the percentage of morphologically mature cells, and increases in
phagocytosis and in lysozyme activity. Differentiation in the melanoma
cells was determined by inhibition of cell growth, formation of den-
dritelike structures, and melanin synthesis. As in the case of the
leukemia cells, induction of differentiation could be detected at low
doses. In analyzing the effect of ten phorbol esters, we found that
their ability to induce terminal differentiation in the HL60 leukemia
cells was correlated with the tumor-promoting activity in mouse skin
(Figure 4). Similar results were found also in the case of the HO
melanoma cells. These results suggest that alteration of cell differentiation characteristics in some cultured cells may represent an approach by which environmental tumor-promoting agents can be studied
and perhaps detected. Thus, future developments in cultured mammalian
cells, including human cells, may allow us to study and identify chemicals with a potential to initiate and/or promote tumor formation in
experimental animals and humans.

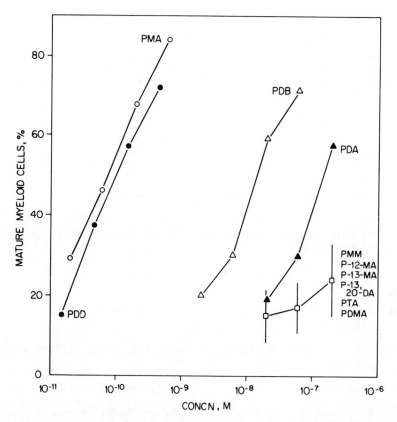

Figure 4. Differentiation in the HL60 cells 2 days after treatment with various concentrations of the phorbol esters. The percentage of mature myeloid cells was determined after cells were stained with Wright/Giemsa. The control cultures contained about 15% mature mye-loid cells. Symbols: o , PMA; • , phorbol-12,13-didecanoate; △ , phorbol-12,13-dibutyrate; ▲ , phorbol-12,13-diacetate; □ , phorbol-12-monomyristate, phorbol-12-monoacetate, phorbol-13-monoacetate, phorbol-13,20-diacetate, phorbol-12,13,-20-triacetate, and phorbol-20-oxo-20-deoxy-12-myristate-13-acetate (From Huberman and Callaham [62]).

ACKNOWLEDGMENTS

This research was sponsored jointly by the National Cancer Institute, under Interagency Agreement 40-636-77, the Environmental Protection Agency, under Interagency Agreement 79-D-X0533, and the Office of

Health and Environmental Research, United States Department of Energy, under contract W-7405-eng-26 with the Union Carbide Corporation.

Dr. Jones is a Postdoctoral Investigator supported by subcontract 3322 from the Biology Division of Oak Ridge Laboratory to the University of Tennessee.

REFERENCES

1. Doll, R., *Nature (London)*, *265*:589-596 (1977).

2. Hiatt, H. H., Watson, J. D., and Winsten, J. A. (eds.), Origins of Human Cancer, Cold Spring Harbor Laboratory, Cold Spring Harbor, New York, 1977.

3. Miller, F. C., and Miller, J. A., *Pharmacol. Rev., 18*:805-838 (1966).

4. Brookes, P., and Lawley, P. D., *Nature (London), 202*:781-784 (1964).

5. Kuroki, T., and Heidelberger, C., *Cancer Res., 31*:2168-2176 (1971).

6. Huberman, E., and Sachs, L., *Int. J. Cancer, 19*:122-127 (1977).

7. Essigmann, J. M., Croy, R. G., Nadzan, A. M., Busby, W. F., Reinhold, V. N., Buchi, G., and Wogan, G. N., *Proc. Natl. Acad. Sci., U.S.A., 74*:1870-1874 (1977).

8. Jeffrey, A. M., Weinstein, I. B., Jenette, K. W., Grzeskowiak, K., Nakahishi, K., Harvey, R. G., Autrup, M., and Harris, C., *Nature (London), 269*:348-350 (1977).

9. Ames, B. N., *Science, 204*:587-593 (1979).

10. Huberman, E., *J. Environ. Pathol. Toxicol., 2*:29-42 (1978).

11. Todaro, G. J., and Huebner, R. J., *Proc. Natl. Acad. Sci., U.S.A., 69*:1009-1015 (1972).

12. Yamamoto, T., Rabinowitz, Z., and Sachs, L., *Nature (London) New Biol., 243*:247-250 (1973).

13. Temin, H. M., *Cancer Res., 34*:2835-2841 (1974).

14. Huberman, E., Mager, R., and Sachs, L., *Nature (London), 264*:360-361 (1976).

15. Chu, E. H. Y., and Malling, H. V., *Proc. Natl. Acad. Sci.*, *U.S.A.*, *61*:1306-1312 (1968).

16. Kao, F. T., and Puck, T. T., *J. Cell. Physiol.*, *78*:139-144 (1971).

17. Huberman, E., and Sachs, L., *Int. J. Cancer*, *13*:326-333 (1974).

18. Newbold, R. F., Wigley, C. B., Thompson, M. H., and Brookes, P., *Mutat. Res.*, *43*:101-116 (1977).

19. Clive, D., Johnson, K. O., Spector, J. F. S., Batson, A. G. and Brown, M. M. M., *Mutat. Res.*, *59*:61-108 (1979).

20. Baker, R. M., Brunette, D. M., Mankovitz, R., Thompson, L. H., Whitmore, G. F., Siminovitch, L., and Till, J. E., *Cell*, *1*:9-21 (1974).

21. Arlett, C. F., Turnbull, C., Harcourt, S. A., Lehmann, A. R., and Collela, C. M., *Mutation Res.*, *33*:261-278 (1975).

22. Miller, J. A., *Cancer Res.*, *39*:559-576 (1970).

23. Heidelberger, C., *Ann. Rev. Biochem.*, *44*:79-121 (1970).

24. Corbett, T. H., Heidelberger, C., and Dove, W. F., *Mol. Pharmacol.* *6*:667-679 (1970).

25. Miller, E. C., and Miller, J. A., In Chemical Mutagens: Principles and Methods for their Detection, Vol. 1, Plenum Press, New York, 1971, pp. 83-119.

26. Gelboin, H. V., Huberman, E., and Sachs, L., *Proc. Natl. Acad. Sci.*, *U.S.A.*, *64*:1188-1194 (1969).

27. Huberman, E., Selkirk, J. K., and Heidelberger, C., *Cancer Res.*, *31*:2161-2167 (1971).

28. Krahn, D. F., and Heidelberger, C., *Mutat. Res.*, *46*:27-44 (1977).

29. Kuroki, T., Drevon, D., and Montesano, R., *Cancer Res.*, *37*:1044-1050 (1977).

30. Mazzaccaro, A., *Mutat. Res.*, *46*:365-373 (1977).

31. Selkirk, J. K., *J. Toxicol. Environ. Health*, *2*:1245-1258 (1977).

32. Bigger, C. A. H., Tomaszewski, J. E., and Dipple, A., *Biochem. Biophys. Res. Commun.*, *80*:229-235 (1978).

33. Jones, C. A., and Huberman, E., *Cancer Res.*, *40*:406-411 (1980).

34. Huberman, E., and Sachs, L., *Proc. Natl. Acad. Sci., U.S.A.,* 73:188-192 (1976).

35. Langenbach, R., Freed, H. J., and Huberman, E., *Proc. Natl. Acad. Sci., U.S.A., 75*:2864-2867 (1978).

36. Huberman, E., Yamaski, H., and Sachs, L., *Int. J. Cancer, 18*:76-83 (1976).

37. Slaga, T. J., Huberman, E., Selkirk, J. K., Harvey, R. G., and Bracken, W. M., *Cancer Res., 38*:1699-1704 (1978).

38. Huberman, E., Sachs, L., Yang, S. K., and Gelboin, H. V., *Proc. Natl. Acad. Sci., U.S.A., 73*:607-611 (1976b).

39. Huberman, E., Yang, S. K., McCourt, D. W., and Gelboin, H. V., *Cancer Lett., 4*:35-43 (1978).

40. Huberman, E., and Slaga, T., *Cancer Res., 39*:411-414 (1979).

41. Huberman, E., Chou, M. W., and Yang, S. K., *Proc. Natl. Acad. Sci., U.S.A., 76*:862-866 (1979).

42. Magee, P. N., Montesano, R., and Preussmann, R., In Chemical Carcinogens (C. E. Searle, ed.), ACS Monography 173, 1976.

43. Wogan, G. N., In Liver Cell Cancer (H. M. Cameron, D. A. Linsell, and Warwick, G. P., eds.), Elsevier-North-Holland Biomedical, New York, 1976, pp. 121-151.

44. San, R. H. C., and Williams, G. M., *Proc. Soc. Exp. Biol. Med., 156*:534-538 (1977).

45. Fry, J. R., Jones, C. A., Wiebkin, P., Bellemann, P., and Bridges, J. W., *Analyt. Biochem., 71*:341-350 (1976).

46. Bartsch, H., Malaveille, C., Camus, A.-M., Brun, G., and Hautefeuille, A., In: Short-Term Mutagenicity Test Systems for Detecting Carcinogens (K. Norpoth and C. Garner, eds.), Springer Verlag, New York, 1979.

47. Druckery, H., Preussmann, R., Ivankovic, S., and Schmahl, D., *Z. Krebsforsch., 69*:103-201 (1967).

48. *IARC Monograph Series, 3*:91-136 (1973).

49. Langenbach, R., Freed, H. Y., Raveh, D., and Huberman, E., *Nature, 276*:277-280 (1978).

50. Jones, C. A., Santella, R., Huberman, E., Selkirk, J. K., and Grunberger, D., submitted to Cancer Research.

51. Berenblum, I., *Prog. Exp. Tumor Res.*, *11*:21-30 (1969).

52. Hecker, E., In: Mechanisms of Tumor Promotion and Cocarcinogenesis
     (T. J. Slaga, A. J. Sivak, and R. Boutwell, eds.), Raven Press,
     New York, 1978, pp. 11-49.

53. Boutwell, R. L., In: Mechanisms of Tumor Promotion and Cocarcino-
     genesis (T. J. Slaga, A. J. Sivak, and R. M. Boutwell, eds.),
     Raven Press, New York, 1978, pp. 49-58.

54. Slaga, T. J., Fischer, S. M., Nelson, K., and Gleason, G. L.,
     Proc. Natl. Acad. Sci., *U.S.A.*, *77*:3659-3663 (1980).

55. McCann, J., and Ames, B. N., In: Origins of Human Cancer (H. H.
     Hiatt, J. D. Watson and J. A. Winston, eds.), Cold Spring Harbor
     Laboratory, Cold Spring Harbor, New York, 1977, pp. 1431-1450.

56. Cohen, R., Pacific, M., Rubinstein, N., Beihl, J., and Holtzer,
     M., *Nature (London)*, *259*:1232-1233 (1976).

57. Rovera, G., O'Brien, T., and Diamond, L., *Proc. Natl. Acad. Sci.*,
     U.S.A., *74*:2894-2896 (1977).

58. Yamasaki, H., Fibach, E., Nudel, U., Weinstein, I. B., Rifkind,
     R. A., and Marks, P. A., *Proc. Natl. Acad. Sci.*, *U.S.A.*, *74*:3451-
     3456 (1977).

59. Ishi, D. N., Fibach, E., Yamasaki, H., and Weinstein, B. I.,
     Science, *200*:556-559 (1978).

60. Diamond, L., O'Brien, T. G., and Rovera, G., *Nature (London)*,
     269:247-249 (1977).

61. Miao, R. M., Fieldsteel, A. H., and Fodge, D., *Nature (London)*,
     274:271-274 (1978).

62. Huberman, E., and Callaham, M. F., *Proc. Natl. Acad. Sci.*, *U.S.A.*,
     76:1293-1297 (1979).

63. Huberman, E., Heckman, C., and Langenbach, R., *Cancer Res.*, *39*:
     2618-2624 (1979).

UNIFYING MECHANISMS IN CARCINOGENESIS

TRANSFORMATION OF CLONED MAMMARY EPITHELIAL CELLS FOLLOWING COMBINED TREATMENT WITH MOUSE MAMMARY TUMOR VIRUS AND DIMETHYLBENZ(A)ANTHRACENE

David K. Howard

Life Sciences Division
Meloy Laboratories, Inc.
Springfield, Virginia

Jeffrey Schlom

National Cancer Institute
National Institute of Health
Bethesda, Maryland

Paul B. Fisher

Department of Microbiology
Institute of Cancer Research
College of Physicians and Surgeons
Columbia University
New York, New York

SUMMARY

We have evaluated the effect of mouse mammary tumor virus (MMTV) and 7,12-dimethylbenz(a)anthracene (DMBA), either alone or in combination on mammary epithelial cells in-vitro. A single-cell clone was derived from the normal mouse mammary gland epithelial cell line, C57MG; it is designated C57MG(clone 2) and is of murine origin as indicated by karyotyping, isoenzyme analyses, and by immunofluorescence analyses using species-specific antisera. This clone failed to induce tumors in syngeneic (C57BL) or athymic (nude) mice. The epithelial origin of the cells was demonstrated by the presence of desmosomes, tono-fibrils and secretory granules. C57MG(clone 2) cells were infected with the MMTV host-range variant MMTV(RIII)vp4, and both infected and mock infected cell cultures were treated with DMBA. Cultures treated with both virus and carcinogen exhibited morphological changes and a slight increase in ability to grow in soft agar after five to seven subcultures. The most striking alteration in the phenotype of cells exposed to the combination of MMTV and DMBA, however, was an increase in their tumorigenic potential in athymic mice. Cultures treated with virus alone or DMBA alone did not show an increase in tumorigenicity. This cell-culture model system may now permit analyses of the crucial molecular events involved in mammary cell transformation.

125

INTRODUCTION

Mammary carcinogenesis in mice is a complex process involving the initiation and progression of preneoplastic lesions, and is influenced
by a variety of agents including ionizing radiation, hormones, chemical
carcinogens, and viruses [1-5]. Although both chemical carcinogens
and mouse mammary tumor viruses (MMTVs) are able to induce preneoplastic lesions in mice, the efficiency of these induction processes can
be altered by changing the hormonal balance of the animals [6,7].
In addition, other factors such as stress, diet, and genetic factors
may play a role in the etiology of murine mammary cancer.

There are several examples in which chemical carcinogens and
either DNA tumor viruses [8-11] or RNA tumor viruses [12-15] can act
synergistically in cell transformation. Current evidence indicates
that chemical carcinogens act by covalently binding to DNA and other
cellular macromolecules and that such interactions induce somatic cell
mutations and/or alterations in gene expression (for review see Refs.
16,17). The frequent association of type-C RNA tumor viruses with
chemically induced transformation [18-20] in rodent systems has led
to speculation that transformation by chemical carcinogens may involve
derepression of oncogenic viruses. On the other hand, it appears that
chemical carcinogens can cause transformation in the absence of detectable virus production [21]. The precise mechanisms of synergy between
viruses and chemicals remain to be elucidated. Recently, Medina et al.
[22] have studied the synergistical interaction of the potent carcinogen 7,12-dimethylbenz(a)anthracene (DMBA) and MMTV in murine mammary
tumorigenesis in the intact mouse. This approach, however, is difficult to interpret at the cellular level because of the complex intermediate events between administration of the carcinogen and the appearance of tumors, and by the possible influence of host factors on the
transformation process. In the series of experiments reported here,
we have developed an in-vitro system to study the interaction of DMBA
and MMTV with murine mammary epithelial cells. We have shown that
treatment of normal mammary epithelial cells with both DMBA and MMTV
results in transformation of the cells, as indicated by increased

tumorigenicity in athymic (nude) mice, increased ability to grow in
semi-solid medium, and the appearance of morphological changes.

MATERIALS AND METHODS

Cells

The preparation and characterization of primary cell cultures from
normal mammary glands of rats has been previously described [23].
Briefly, partial collagenase digestion and Ficoll gradient sedimentation facilitated the separation of epithelial elements derived from
mammary glands of perphenazine stimulated normal virgin rats. In addition to morphological features, the rat normal mammary gland cultures
were characteristic of mammary cells in that they produced alpha-
lactalbumin as detected by specific radioimmunoassay [23]. These cells
when examined in our laboratory (by C. M. Calberg-Bacq, University of
Liege, Belgium) were shown to contain desmosomes, tonofibrils, and
microvilli, confirming their epithelial origin.

The C57BL/6 murine mammary gland cell line, C57MG [24], was obtained from Dr. E. Lasfargues, Institute for Medical Research, Camden,
NJ. This line was cloned at passage 31. The cells used for in-vitro
virus-chemical cocarcinogenesis studies were one of the resulting single cell clones, designated C57MG(clone 2). The NMuMG cell line,
derived from mammary glands of an adult Namru mouse [25] was obtained
from Dr. A. Hackett, Naval Biomedical Research Laboratories, Oakland,
CA. All cell lines were tested for species of origin by isoenzyme
analyses, karyotyping, and immunofluorescence analyses, and were shown
to be of the proper species of origin. These tests for species of
origin were performed through the Office of Program and Logistics,
Biological Carcinogenesis Branch, National Cancer Institute.

Virus and Infection of Cells

The MMTV host-range variants, MMTV(C3H)vp4 and MMTV(RIII)vp4, were
isolated by four serial virus passages in feline CrFK cells as previ
ously described [26]. Virions obtained from 24 hr collections of cell
culture supernatant fluids from infected CrFK cells were concentrated

by isopycnic gradient centrifugation in sucrose gradients as previously described [27]. Several preparations of virus were pooled and filtered through a 0.45 um Millipore filter, pre-coated with polyvinylpyrrolidone [28] to remove any contaminating bacteria. The amount of virus in these stock solutions was determined by using group-specific radioimmunoassays for the 52,000d major external glycoprotein (gp52) and the 28,000d major internal protein (p28) of MMTVs, as previously described [29,30]. Aliquots of viruses were then stored over liquid nitrogen to provide stocks of virus for reproducible infection of cells.

The method for infecting cells with MMTVs has been previously described in detail [31,32]. Briefly, the procedure was as follows: cells were seeded in 75 cm^2 flasks at known cell densities and virus was added 24 hrs later in medium containing 4 ug per ml polybrene. Twenty-four or 48 hrs later, the medium was changed to medium without polybrene. At appropriate intervals thereafter, 24 hr collections of culture medium were assayed for the presence of progeny virus using a group-specific radioimmunoassay for MMTV gp52, as previously described [29].

Toxicity of DMBA

To determine the concentration of DMBA to be used in virus-chemical cocarcinogenesis experiments, the toxicity of various concentrations of DMBA for C57MG(clone 2) cells was measured. Approximately 2×10^6 C57MG(clone 2) cells were seeded in 100 mm cell culture plates and treated 24 hrs later with 0.005 to 5 ug per ml of DMBA. After treatment for 24 hrs, the carcinogen-containing medium was removed and the cells were washed with sterile phosphate-buffered saline. Control cultures were treated with either 0.1% dimethylsulfoxide (DMSO, carcinogen solvent) or with growth medium for 24 hrs. The cultures were then trypsinized and 3×10^2 cells were plated in each of five 100 mm cell culture plates to determine their plating efficiency. Cultures were refed twice per week with fresh growth medium and stained with Giemsa after 10 to 14 days. The number of colonies was then counted.

Virus-Chemical Cocarcinogenesis

C57MG(clone 2) cells were seeded at a density of 1×10^5 cells per 75 cm^2 flask and infected with MMTV(RIII)vp4 24 hrs later at a multiplicity of infection of 1×10^5 particles per cell. Mock-infected cultures were set up in parallel. Forty-eight hours after infection, both infected and mock-infected cells were treated for 24 hrs with 1 ug per ml DMBA, or with the DMSO solvent. Cultures were then washed twice in sterile phosphate buffered saline and refed with fresh growth medium. Thereafter, cultures were passaged upon reaching confluency, at approximately weekly intervals.

Transformation Assays

To determine the tumorigenic potential of cultures in-vivo, cells were inoculated into BALB/c athymic (nude) mice. Cells were inoculated subcutaneously at a concentration of 2×10^6 cells in 0.2 ml of serum-free medium. Animals were examined weekly for the appearance of tumors.

The ability of cells to grow in semi-solid agar was also determined. Cells were suspended in 0.4% Difco Bacto Agar in growth medium and 5×10^4 cells in this suspension were overlaid onto 5 ml of 0.8% agar in 60 mm cell culture plates. Cultures were incubated in a humidified incubator at 37°C in an atmosphere of 5% CO_2 for 14 to 21 days. Colonies of diameter greater than 0.2 mm were counted.

Electron Microscopy

C57MG(clone 2) cells were grown in 5 cm^2 plastic coverslips in disposable Leighton tubes until they reached confluence. The culture medium was removed and the cells rinsed once with ice-cold cacodylate buffer (0.1 M sodium cacodylate in distilled water, pH 7.0). The cells were then fixed for 2 hrs at 4°C with 2% gluteraldehyde in cacodylate buffer and rinsed twice at 4°C with cacodylate buffer, each rinse being for 30 min. The cells were post-fixed in 1% osmium tetroxide, washed

for 1 to 2 hr in distilled water, stained with 2% uranyl acetate in
50% ethanol, dehydrated in ethanol-propylene oxide and embedded in
Epon-Araldite. Transverse sections were stained with uranyl acetate
and lead citrate and examined in a Siemans-Elmiskop 1A electron microscope.

RESULTS

Mammary Gland Cell Cultures

Comparisons of the properties of mammary tumor cells in culture with
those of normal mammary gland epithelial cells have been hampered by
the paucity of continuous cell lines of normal mammary gland epithelial
cells. For several decades attempts have been made to culture mammary
epithelial cells free of fibroblasts and adipose cells, but until recently these efforts have had only limited success. Recently, Wicha
et al. [23] described a technique for the preparation of epithelial
cell cultures from the mammary glands of rats. Using this technique,
we have successfully established mammary gland epithelial cell cultures
from a number of rat and mouse strains. We have been able to maintain
these cultures for up to eight passages in-vitro.

We have also derived single-cell clones from the normal mouse
mammary gland cell line, designated C57MG [24]. One of these single-
cell clones, C57MG(clone 2), has been characterized in some detail.
The cells exhibit a typical epithelial cell morphology with polygonal
cells forming a characteristic "cobblestone" monolayer (Figure 3a).
When examined in the electron microscope, these cells have clearly
identifiable desmosomes and tonofibrils (Figure 1). As expected, they
also contain secretory granules, since one function of mammary gland
epithelial cells is to secrete materials into the lumina of the ducts
of the mammary glands. When inoculated into either syngeneic C57BL/6
or athymic (nude) mice, these cells failed to induce any tumors during
an observation period of 50 to 60 days (Table 1). In comparison, the
mouse mammary gland cell line, NMuMG, induced benign cysts in athymic

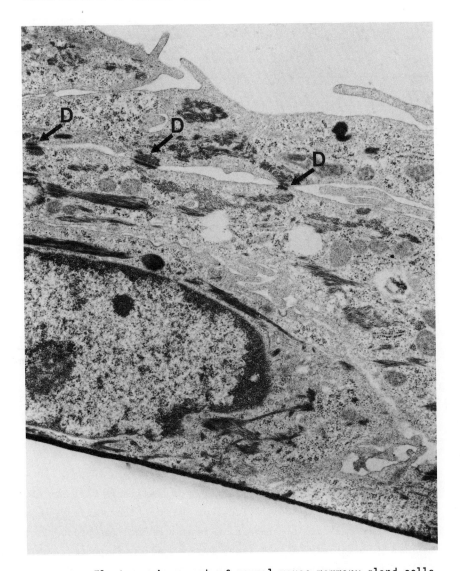

Figure 1. Electron micrograph of normal mouse mammary gland cells in culture. C57MG(clone 2) cells were grown on plastic coverslips until they reached confluence. The cells were then rinsed in ice-cold cacodylate buffer, fixed with 2% glutaraldehyde in this buffer, and the coverslips embedded in Epon. After dehydration and staining, the cell sheet was sectioned vertically and examined in the electron microscope. The arrows indicate the location of desmosomes, (D). The magnifiaction is X35,000.

TABLE 1
Tumorigenic Potential of Mammary Gland Cells
in Athymic (Nude) and Syngeneic Mice

| Cell Line | Dose/Route | No. Mice with Tumor/Total No. | |
		Athymic (Nude)	C57BL/6N
C57MG, P31	2 X 10^6/S.Q.	0/8	0/5
C57MG(clone 2), p13	2 X 10^6/S.Q.	0.8	0/10
NMuMG, P17	2 X 10^6/S.Q.	1/5[a]	N.T.
Mm5mt/c_1, P29	2 X 10^6/S.Q.	5/5	N.T.

Cells were inoculated subcutaneously into athymic (nude) mice or syngeneic C57BL/6N mice at a concentration of 2 X 10^6 cells in 0.2 ml of serum-free culture medium. Mice were examined at weekly intervals for the appearance of tumors. The experiment was terminated 154 days after the inoculation of cells.

[a]Well differentiated, benign cystic growth.
N.T. = Not tested.

(nude) mice, confirming earlier findings [25]. Thus, the C57MG(clone 2) cell are of epithelial origin, as evidenced by the presence of desmosomes and tonofibrils, and "normal" as indicated by their inability to induce tumors in syngeneic or athymic (nude) mice.

Infection of Cells with MMTVs

Recently, we have reported the isolation of host-range variants of MMTVs [26]. In comparison to wild-type MMTVs, which replicate only in feline and mink cells, these host-range variants can productively infect a wide variety of cell lines from a number of species (Table 2). The MMTV host-range variants are capable of productively infecting a total of twelve cell lines from six different species. As seen in Table 2 both host-range variants can productively infect a number of primary cultures and established cell lines of normal mammary gland cells from feline, murine, and rat species. Cultures from normal mammary glands of Wistar-Furth, Wistar-Lewis, ACI and F344 (Fischer) rats

TABLE 2
Host-Range of MMTV Variants

Species	Cell Line Designation	Tissue of Origin	Days to Initial Virus Production	
			MMTV(RIII)vp4	MMTV(C3H)vp4
Mouse	NIH-3T3	Embryo	39	53
	NMuMG	Mammary gland of Namru mouse	13	16
	C57BL	Mammary gland of C57BL mouse	36	30
Rat	FRE	Embryo	24	50
	Secondary Embryo	Embryo	33	>62
	Normal rat mammary gland	Mammary gland	33	25
Cat	CrFK	Embryo kidney	5	6
	Normal mammary gland	Mammary gland	67	75
Dog	Cf2Th	Thymus	24	45
Human	HP574	Full-term placenta	26	28
Bat	Tb1Lu	Lung	>83	47

Twenty-four hour collections of supernatant culture fluids from confluent 75 cm^2 flasks were assayed after infection at 7-10 day intervals using a group-specific radioimmunoassay for MMTV gp52.

TABLE 3
Infection of Primary Rat Mammary Gland Cultures with
MMTV Host-Range Variants

Rat Strain	Day First Positive	Maximum Virus Production(ng)
ACI - Experiment 1	33	220
ACI - Experiment 2	43	90
ACI - Experiment 3	12	2,800
Wistar-Lewis	19	1,000
Wistar-Furth	32	190
F344	112	180

Primary cultures of rat mammary gland cells were infected with MMTV-
(RIII)vp4. Supernatant fluids were collected at approximately weekly
intervals and virus in the fluid was pelleted at 196,000 X g for 60
minutes through 2.5 ml of 20% glycerol. Pellets were resuspended and
the virus content quantitated in a group-specific radioimmunoassay
for MMTV gp52.

were permissive for productive infection by a MMTV host-range variant
(Table 3). MMTV-infected rat mammary gland cultures have been maintained up to three months with persistent virus production.

C57MG(clone 2) cells were readily susceptible to infection with
the MMTV host-range variant, MMTV(RIII)vp4 (Table 4). At a multiplicity of infection of 1×10^5 particles per cell, de-novo progeny virus
could be detected in cell culture supernatant fluids with as short a
latent period as 4 to 5 days. These cells continued to release progeny
virus during an observation period of almost 100 days. In comparison,
C57MG(clone 3) cells were totally refractory to productive infection
by MMTV(RIII)vp4 while C57MG(clone 1) cells were transiently infected,
with progeny virus being detected only between approximately day 10
and day 15 after infection.

The use of primary cultures of mammary gland cells for virus-
chemical cocarcinogenesis studies has inherent problems. It is difficult to obtain reproducible results with cultures derived from different animals (Table 3), and, in addition, it is difficult to know which
subpopulations of cells in these uncloned cultures is responsible for

TABLE 4
Infection of C57MG Single Cell Clones with MMTV

Days Post Infection	Titer of MMTV in Supernatant Culture Fluids (ng)		
	Clone 1	Clone 2	Clone 3
0	0	0	0
9	8	40	0
14	10	56	0
22	0	167	0
50	0	417	0
78	0	294	0

Cells were seeded at 1 X 10^5 cells per 75 cm^2 flask. Twenty-four hours later, MMTV(RIII)vp4 at a multiplicity of infection of 1 X 10^5 particles per cell, was added in culture medium containing 4 ug per ml polybrene. Supernatant fluids were harvested at the times indicated and virus in the fluid was pelleted at 196,000 X g for 60 minutes through 2.5 ml of 20% glycerol in a Beckman SW4] rotor. Pellets were resuspended and the amount of virus present quantitated in a group-specific radioimmunoassay for MMTV gp52.

effects seen with the addition of virus or chemical. For these reasons, we chose to perform virus-chemical cocarcinogenesis studies using the cloned mouse mammary gland epithelial cell line C57MG(clone 2).

Oncogenicity of MMTV Host-Range Variants

Since MMTV host-range variants were of interest for in-vitro transformation assays, their tumorigenic potential in-vivo was determined. BALB/c mice were chosen as the host animals due to their previously reported susceptibility to MMTV replication and oncogenicity [33]. Twenty-four hour harvests of MMTV(C3H), obtained from the supernatant cell culture fluids of the Mm5mt/c_1 mammary tumor cell line, and MMTV-(C3H)vp4, obtained from CrFK feline cells, were purified and concentrated in an identical manner [31]. The quantity of MMTV virions in each preparation was calculated on the basis of radioimmunoassay for both MMTV gp52 and p28. Various doses of each preparation were inocu-

lated intraperitoneally into 6 to 8 week old female BALB/c mice which
were subsequently force-bred. The incidence of spontaneous mammary
tumors in this colony is approximately 10% at one year of age. This
incidence was also observed in mice inoculated with the diluent. An
increase in mammary tumor incidence was observed over inoculation doses
ranging from 10^5 to 10^8 particles for both wild-type and host range
variant MMTVs. Inoculation of as little as 10^4 MMTV(C3H)vp4 particles
resulted in mammary tumors in 41% of the mice.

The RNA genomes of MMTVs of high oncogenic potential obtained
from C3H, RIII and GR mice have all been shown to contain a subset of
sequences that is found in the DNAs of early mammary tumors of these
mice [27]. These sequences are also retained in the host-range variants of MMTVs. Drohan and Schlom [34] have demonstrated that these
sequences, termed tumor associated sequences (TAS), are not found,
however, in either the DNA of normal BALB/c tissues or in the DNA of
spontaneous BALB/c mammary tumors. Some of the mammary tumors resulting from the inoculation of MMTV(C3H) and MMTV(C3H)vp4 were examined
for the presence of TAS provirus. Tumors resulting from the inoculation of as little as 10^4 particles of MMTV(C3H)vp4 containing TAS
provirus in their DNA, whereas spontaneous mammary tumors from BALB/c
mice did not contain these sequences. Therefore, a MMTV host range
variant that has increased its ability to replicate in-vitro by several
orders of magnitude has still maintained its oncogenic potential.

Toxicity of DMBA for C57MG(Clone 2) Cells

The plating efficiency of C57MG(clone 2) cells was determined after
treatment of replicate cultures of cells with various concentrations
of DMBA or with the carcinogen solvent, dimethysulfoxide. The plating
efficiency of cells treated with either culture medium or with DMSO
was 22%. Addition of DMBA at concentrations between 0.005 and 0.1 ug
per ml had no effect on the plating efficiency of the cells (Figure
2). Addition of higher concentrations of DMBA, however, reduced the
plating efficiency of the cells. The plating efficiency was reduced
to approximately 20% of control cultures by the addition of 5 ug per

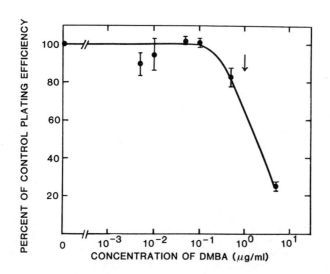

Figure 2. Effect of 7,12-dimethylbenz(a)anthracene on the plating efficiency of C57MG(clone 2) cells. C57MG(clone 2) cells were seeded at a density of 2 X 10⁶ cells per 100 mm plastic tissue culture plate and replicate cultures were treated 24 hours later with the indicated concentration of 7,12-dimethylbenz(a)anthracene in 0.05% dimethylsulfoxide. After 24 hours, the cells were washed three times in phosphate buffered saline, trypsinized, counted and 300 cells seeded in each of five tissue culture plates. After 10-14 days, when macroscopic cell colonies were visible, the cells were fixed with 10% formaldehyde, stained with Giemsa and the colonies were counted.

ml DMBA (Figure 2). For further studies we chose to use a concentration of 1 ug per ml DMBA. At this concentration, the plating efficiency of C57MG(clone 2) cells was reduced to approximately 80-85% of that obtained with control cultures.

Virus-Chemical Cocarcinogenesis

C57MG(clone 2) cells were infected with the host range variant MMTV-(RIII)vp4, and both infected and uninfected cultures were treated with 1 ug per ml DMBA or with DMSO. The most dramatic change in the phenotype of cells following treatment with both virus and DMBA was a marked increase in their tumorigenic potential in athymic (nude) mice when compared to either control cultures (uninfected cultures treated with DMSO) or with cultures treated with virus or DMBA alone (Table 5). This increase in tumorigenicity was first observed after five passages

TABLE 5
Inoculation of C57MG(Clone 2) Mammary Gland Cells
Into Athymic (Nude) Mice

Passage Level After Treatment	No. of Animals with Tumors/Total No. Animals			
	Control	Virus	DMBA	Virus + DMBA
P1	0/20	0/20	0/20	0/20
P3	0/8	0/8	0/8	0/8
P5	1/16	1/16	0/16	6/16
P7	0/8	0/8	0/8	3/8

C57MG(clone 2) cells were treated with various combinations of 7,12-
dimethylbenz(a)anthracene and MMTV. At every second passage after
treatment, cells were inoculated into athymic (nude) mice. Cells
were inoculated subcutaneously at a concentration of 2 X 10^6 cells
in 0.2 ml of serum-free medium. The appearance of tumors was observed
for a period of 12 to 14 weeks.

in-vitro and was still seen after seven passages in-vitro. In addition
to the observed increased in tumorigenicity, clearly discernable morphological changes were seen in cultures treated with both virus and
chemical when compared to control cultures or to cultures treated with
either agent alone. Cells treated with both virus and chemical grew
with a random orientation and the appearance of numerous long, thin
pseudopodia was noted (Figure 3d). Cells treated only with DMBA also
exhibited these morphologic properties but to a lesser degree (Figure
3c). Control cultures and cultures treated only with virus showed
little or no evidence of random cell orientation or the presence of
pseudopodia and were indistinguishable from each other (Figure 3a, b).

Cultures of treated and untreated cells were suspended in semi-
solid agar to determine their ability to form colonies in this medium.
Control cultures grew at a low efficiency when suspended in 0.4% agar,
with a cloning efficiency of approximately 0.27%. Treatment with
virus, DMBA, or with both agents, resulted in a slight increase in
the ability of cells to grow in semi-solid medium, yielding 0.55%
colony forming efficiency. This phenomonen, as well as the morphologi-

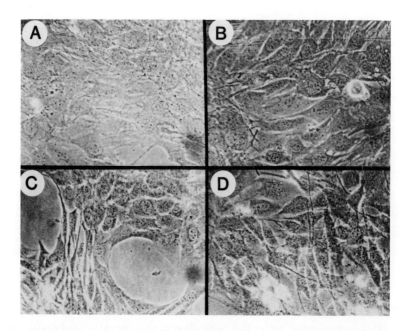

Figure 3. Light microscopy of C57MG(clone 2) cells following treatment with MMTV and DMBA. C57MG(clone 2) cells were infected with
MMTV(RIII)vp4 and both infected and mock-infected cultures were treated
with DMBA. Morphological changes in the cultures were first seen at
passage 5. (A) Uninfected C57MG(clone 2) cells treated with the carcinogen solvent, dimethysulfoxide; (B) C57MG(clone 2) cells infected
with MMTV(RIII)vp4 and treated with the carcinogen solvent, DMSO; (C)
Uninfected cells treated with 1 ug per ml DMBA; (D) MMTV(RIII)vp4 infected C57MG(clone 2) cells treated with DMBA.

cal changes, first occurred after approximately five passages in-vitro,
coinciding with the appearance of an increased tumorigenic potential
of the treated cells.

DISCUSSION

Until recently, three major obstacles have prevented the development
of an in-vitro model for virus-mediated mammary cell transformation.
These are, (1) the inability to infect cells in culture with MMTVs;
(2) the inability to generate, passage and maintain well-characterized
cultures of normal, mammary epithelial cell substrates; (3) the lack
of reliable in-vitro assays for identifying transformed mammary gland
epithelial cells.

Lasfargues et al. [28,35,36] and Howard et al. [31] have demonstrated the ability of the highly oncogenic MMTVs of C3H, RIII and GR
mice to productively infect feline and mink cells in-vitro. Establishment of these infections, however, required extremely high multiplicities of infection and latent periods of up to three months for the
appearance of de-novo progeny virus. Recently, we have reported [26]
the isolation of host-range variants of MMTVs that productively infect
feline cells with extremely high efficiency (at multiplicities of infection of less than 1 particle per cell and with latent periods of
as short as four days). In addition, whereas wild-type MMTVs can infect only mink and feline cells, these host-range variants productively
infect a wide variety of cells lines from a number of different species. These host-range variants also retained their oncogenic potential in-vivo. The availability of these host-range variants of MMTVs
has thus removed the first obstacle to the development of an in-vitro
model for virus-mediated mammary gland epithelial cell transformation.

Techniques have recently been described for the isolation and
characterization of primary cultures from normal mammary glands of
rats [23]. In addition, at least one normal cell line of mouse mammary gland epithelial cells, designated C57MG [24], and one mouse cell
line (NMuMG) with characteristics of premalignant mammary gland epithelium [25], are now widely available. Using the techniques described
by Wicha et al. [23], we have also been able to prepare and maintain
cell cultures from feline mammary glands [32] and we have shown that
primary mammary gland epithelial cell cultures of murine, feline, and
rat origin, as well as the C57MG and NMuMG established cell lines, can
be productively infected with MMTV host-range variants [32]. Together
with our ability to maintain primary mammary gland cell cultures for
at least eight passages in-vitro, these recent advances in the art
of generating mammary gland cultures now provide suitable cell systems
for the development of in-vitro mammary gland epithelial cell transformation models.

The third prerequisite for the development of in-vitro transformation models for virus-mediated mammary tumorigenesis is a reliable
assay that distinguishes between normal and malignant mammary epitheli-

al cells. There is no simple, quantitative, reliable parameter for
in-vitro assay of transformed epithelial cells (for review, see Ref.
37). Butel et al. [38] have examined a number of mouse mammary tumor
cell lines for in-vitro growth parameters which correlate with tumorigenicity in-vivo. Their findings indicate that there was no growth
parameter in-vitro which consistently correlated with tumorigenicity
in-vivo. Epithelial cells cultured from normal, preneoplastic, and
neoplastic mammary tissues are similar in size and shape, have the
same growth rates and saturation densities in-vitro, adhere tightly
to glass or plastic substrates, and show little tendency to pile up
or overgrow each other [39,40]. Our approach to identifying transformed mammary gland epithelial cells, therefore, has been to identify
such transformed cultures by their ability to induce tumors in athymic
(nude) mice. Once such transformed cultures have been identified, we
hope to then determine which in-vitro properties correlate with their
in-vivo tumorigenicity.

Using host-range variants of MMTVs together with a well-characterized cloned normal mouse mammary epithelial cell line and assaying
for transformation by determining the ability of cell cultures to induce tumors in athymic (nude) mice, we have obtained evidence that
treatment of mammary gland epithelial cells with both MMTV and DMBA
results in the transformation of these cells. Although we observed
a concomitant increase in the ability of the treated cells to grow in
soft agar, untreated cells also showed some growth in agar. It may
now be possible, however, to determine exactly which in-vitro growth
properties of transformed mammary gland cells best correlate with in-
vivo tumorigenicity. This model system will also now provide a means
of studying the interactions of multiple agents (viruses, chemicals,
hormones, tumor promoters, growth factors, and others) in the in-vitro
transformation of mammary gland epithelial cells.

ACKNOWLEDGMENTS

We wish to thank Dr. I. Bernard Weinstein for valuable advice and
discussions. We also wish to acknowledge the able technical assistance
of Allen Scott, Valerie Ahmuty, and Jeanne Mitchell. We thank Dr. W.

Drohan for assistance with molecular hybridization studies to identify virus-induced tumors, Dr. Y. A. Teramoto for assistance in radioimmuno-assay studies, and Dr. P. Horan Hand for assistance in developing primary cultures of mammary gland epithelial cells. Support for these studies was provided in part by the National Cancer Institute, contract NO1-CP-43223.

REFERENCES

1. Bentvelzen, P., *Biophys. Acta, 355*:236-259 (1974).

2. DeOme, K. B., and Nandi, S., In: Viruses Inducing Cancer, (W. J. Burdette, ed.), Univ. Utah Press, Salt Lake City, 1966, pp. 127.

3. Medina, J., *J. Tox. Envirn. Health, 1*:551-560 (1976).

4. Cardiff, R. D., Wellings, S. R., and Faulkin, L. J., *Cancer, 39*:2734-2746 (1977).

5. Weinstein, I. B., In: Cell Biology of Breast Cancer, (M. Brennan, and M. A. Rich, eds.), Academic Press, New York, (in press) (1980).

6. Medina, D., DeOme, K. B., Young, L., *J. Natl. Cancer Inst., 44*: 167-174 (1970).

7. Faulkin, L. J., *J. Natl. Cancer Inst., 36*:289-298 (1966).

8. Casto, B. C., Pieczynski, W. J., and DiPaolo, J. A., *Cancer Res., 34*:72-78 (1974).

9. Coggin, J. H., *J. Virol., 3*:458-462 (1969).

10. Fisher, P. B., Weinstein, I. B., Eisenberg, D., and Ginsberg, H. S., *Proc. Natl. Acad. Sci., U.S.A., 75*:2311-2314 (1978).

11. Fisher, P. B., and Weinstein, I. B., Chemical-viral Interactions and Multistep Aspects of Cell Transformation. In: Molecular and Cellular Aspects of Carcinogen Screening Tests, (R. Montesano, H. Bartsch, and L. Tomatis, eds.), Intl. Agency for Research on Cancer, 1980, pp. 113-131.

12. Freeman, A. E., Weisburger, E. K., Weisburger, J. H., Wolford, R. G., Maryak, J. M., and Huebner, R. J., *J. Natl. Cancer Inst., 51*:799-808 (1973).

13. Rhim, J. S., Vass, W., Cho, H. Y., and Huebner, R. J., *Intl. J. Cancer, 7*:65-74 (1971).

14. Rhim, J. S., Park, D. K., Weisburger, E. K., and Weisburger, J. H., *J. Natl. Cancer Inst.*, *52*:1167-1173 (1974).

15. Price, P. J., Bellow, T. M., King, M. P., Freeman, A. E., Gilden, R. V., and Huebner, R. J., *Proc. Natl. Acad. Sci.*, *U.S.A.*, *73*:152-155 (1976).

16. Heidelberger, C., *Ann. Rev. Biochem.*, *44*:49-121 (1975).

17. Weinstein, I. B., Yamasaki, H., Wigler, M., Lee, L. S., Fisher, P. B., Jeffrey, A., and Grunberger, D., Molecular and Cellular Events Associated with the Action of Initiating Carcinogens and Tumor Promoters. In: Carcinogens: Identification and Mechanisms of Action, (A. C. Griffin, and C. R. Shaw, eds.), Raven Press, New York, 1979, pp. 399-418.

18. Igel, H. J., Huebner, R. J., Turner, H. C., Kotin, P., and Falk, H. L., *Science*, *166*:1624-1626 (1969).

19. Whitmire, C. E., Salemo, R. A., Rabstein, L. S., Huebner, R. J., and Turner, H. C., *J. Natl. Cancer Inst.*, *47*:1255-1265 (1971).

20. Rhim, J. S., Dah, F. G., Cho, H. Y., Elder, E., and Vernon, M. L., *J. Natl. Cancer Inst.*, *50*:255-261 (1973).

21. Rapp, U. R., Nowinski, R. C., Reznikoff, C., and Heidelberger, C., *Virology*, *65*:392-409 (1975).

22. Medina, D., Butel, J. S., Socher, S. H., and Miller, F. L., *Cancer Res.*, *40*:368-373 (1980).

23. Wicha, M. A., Liotta, L. A., and Kidwell, W. R., *Cancer Res.*, *39*:426-435 (1979).

24. Vaidya, A. B., Lasfargues, E. Y., Sheffield, J. B., and Coutinho, W. G., *Virology*, *90*:12-22 (1978).

25. Owens, R. B., Smith, H. S., and Hackett, A. J., *J. Natl. Cancer Inst.*, *53*:261-269 (1974).

26. Howard, D. K., and Schlom, J., *Proc. Natl. Acad. Sci.*, *U.S.A.*, *75*:5718-5722 (1978).

27. Drohan, W., Kettman, R., Colcher, D., and Schlom, J., *J. Virology*, *21*:986-995 (1977).

28. Lasfargues, E. Y., Lasfargues, J. C., Dion, A. S., Greene, A. E., and Moore, D. H., *Cancer Res.*, *36*:67-72 (1976).

29. Teramoto, Y. A., Kufe, D., and Schlom, J., *Proc. Natl. Acad. Sci.*, *U.S.A.*, *74*:3564-3568 (1977).

30. Teramoto, Y. A., and Schlom, J., *Cancer Res.*, *38*:1990-1995 (1978).

31. Howard, D. K., Colcher, D., Teramoto, Y. A., Young, J. M., and Schlom, J., *Cancer Res.*, *37*:2696-2704 (1977).

32. Howard, D. K., and Schlom, J., *J. Gen. Virol.*, *47*:439-448 (1980).

33. Bentvelzen, P., *Intl. Rev. Exp. Pathol.*, *11*:259-297 (1972).

34. Drohan, W., and Schlom, J., *J. Virol.*, *31*:53-62 (1979).

35. Lasfargues, E. Y., Kramarsky, B., Lasfargues, J. C., and Moore, D. H., *J. Natl. Cancer Inst.*, *53*:1831-1833 (1974).

36. Lasfargues, E. Y., Vaidya, A. B., Lasfargues, J. C., and Moore, D. H., *J. Natl. Cancer Inst.*, *57*:447-449 (1976).

37. Weinstein, I. B., Wigler, M., and Stadler, U., Analyses of the Mechanism of Chemical Carcinogenesis in Epithelial Cell Cultures. In: Screening Tests in Chemical Carcinogenesis, (R. Montesano, H. Bartsch and L. Tomatis, eds.), Intl. Agency for Research on Cancer, 1976, pp. 355-381.

38. Butel, J. S., Dudley, J. P., and Medina, D., *Cancer Res.*, *37*:1892-1900 (1977).

39. Pickett, P. B., Pitelka, D. R., Hamamoto, S. T., and Misfeldt, D. S., *J. Cell Biol.*, *66*:316-322 (1975).

40. Voyles, B. A., and McGrath, C. M., *Int. J. Cancer*, *18*:498-509 (1976).

VIRUS-CELL INTERACTIONS DURING HORMONAL CARCINOGENESIS IN BALB/C FEMALE MICE

Charles M. McGrath
Herbert D. Soule
Richard F. Jones

Department of Tumor Biology
Michigan Cancer Foundation
Detroit, Michigan

SUMMARY

Evidence is given which suggests that a replication defective variant of MuMTV, genetically distinguishable from MuMTV-S or viruses activated in Balb/c neoplasms induced by it, is activated in Balb/c mammary neoplasms induced by a hormonal perturbation that causes a non-cyclic hyperplastic proliferation of the mammary parenchyma. Biologic details of this study suggest further that (1) unlike infectious MuMTV-S which acts in tumorigenesis primarily in early precancerous transformations from normal, hormonal perturbation acts primarily in tumorigenic transformations in precancerous tissue; (2) the action of the hormonal perturbation in tumorigenesis is in some ways analogous to promotion, classically defined and is independent of an effect on cell growth rate; (3) the hormonal perturbation that causes mammary neoplasms in Balb/c females is itself insufficient stimulus for induction of the replication-defective MuMTV variant; and (4) the induced structural MuMTV information detected in precancerous Balb/c neoplasms is insufficient stimulus for tumor formation in those neoplasms.

INTRODUCTION

Mammary cancer in mice is generally considered a "viral cancer" and
that model can indeed be found in certain inbred strains like C3H
and RIII [1,2]. Even in these high cancer incidence strains, however,
but especially in their low incidence counterparts, it is clear that
infectious viruses alone cannot account for the origins of mammary
cancer in mice. Host genotype and endocrine status also play major
roles in the onset and development of the disease [3].

We have nonetheless emphasized mammary tumor viruses for study
of mammary cancer origins because of the unique position that they
occupy in ordering the other two major disease influences, genetics
and hormones. In one phase of their life cycle, these viruses are
transmitted as genes integrated in the mouse germ line, which segregate
in mammary cells during hormone-instructed postnatal differentiation
essentially as other differentiation genes [4]. Integrated viral
genes are inducible by certain mammotropic hormones [5] and certain
hormones increase incidence of mammary cancers [6,7]. At issue is
whether these phenomena are cause-effect linked, whether carcinogenic
hormone milieu induce viral information in mammary cells, and if induced viral information acts in the transformation of cells.

A Biological Comparison of "Hormonal" and "Viral"
Mammary Carcinogenesis in Balb/c Mice

There are basically two models in which to study virus-cell interactions in hormonal mammary carcinogenesis in mice. It is important
to note that phenomenonologically these two models differ only in
their emphasis on either viruses or hormones in the neoplastic process.
Both models can be introduced in inbred Balb/c mice, normally a low
mammary cancer incidence inbred strain [2]. This is often done to
normalize the variable influence of host genotype in modulating hormone responses [3].

In one model, the "virus-predominant model", Balb/c females are
infected with a highly oncogenic variant of MuMTV at birth (e.g. MuMTV-

S, which gives Balb/cfC3H). In the other, the "hormone-predominant
model", Balb/c females are endocrinologically manipulated without infection. Several hormone treatments can induce mammary cancers in
both models [2,6,8]. One endocrinologic perturbation that generates
mammary cancers in Balb/c (and other strains, see [9,10]) is translo-
cation of hypophyseal glands from the normal neural hypothalamic connection to other sites in the body. The effect of severing the hypothalamic connection is to inhibit release of luteinizing hormone (LH)
and follicular stimulating hormone (FSH) and to stimulate constitutive
release of prolactin [10]. Prolactin is luteotropic, causing accumulation of corpora lutea in the ovaries, which then secrete progesterone
[9,10].

The effect of hypophyseal isografts (HI) on mammary cancer in
Balb/cfC3H (infected) and Balb/c (uninfected) females is shown in
Figure 1. After some time, cancer incidence reaches 100% in both
models. In our hands, the effect is organ-specific in that cancers
of other organs including ovary and uterus are rarely if ever encountered.

In the virus-predominant model, infectious virus is clearly not
sufficient for tumorigenesis. Without the hormonal challenge of HI
(or pregnancy [2]) only small numbers of tumors develop in infected
females, fewer even than in uninfected, HI-treated groups (Figure 1).
Without HI, virgin Balb/c females in the Michigan Cancer Foundation
colony rarely develop mammary cancer and then only after the second
year of life (Figure 1). Pregnancy has no added effect on that incidence; in fact, there is some data, merely anecdotal presently, that
suggests that multiple pregnancy results in lower mammary cancer incidence in Balb/c females.

While the final mammary tumor incidence reaches 100% in both
models, two differences in natural history are noteworthy. First, all
cancers that develop in Balb/cfC3H are alveolar carcinomas in which
considerable adenomatous organization is retained in neoplastic tissue.
In contrast, all early tumors (those that develop during ca. 7-13
months of hormonal perturbations) are adenoacanthomas, with squamous

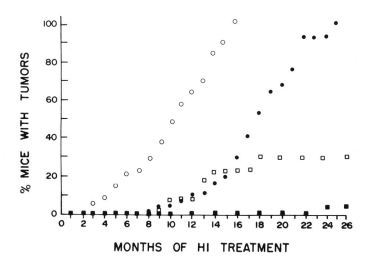

Figure 1. The incidence of Mammary Tumors in Hypophyseal Isografted (HI) Balb/c and Balb/cfC3H Mice. Mice between 3 and 4 weeks of age, which received pituitary isografts under the kidney capsule (O and ●), or were normally cycling non-treated mice (□, ■), were palpated at monthly intervals for appearance of mammary tumors. Open symbols, Balb/cfC3H; closed symbols, Balb/c.

metaplasia (Figure 2). Tumors that develop after ca. 13 months are either adenoacanthomas or carcinomas, the latter tumors, also with considerable adenomatous organization (Figure 2). The significance of this finding is unclear, but may relate to differences in stem cells at risk to "hormonal" and "viral" carcinogenesis [11].

The second major difference in natural history of cancer in the two models is in onset time. Latency is decreased from ca. 8 months in the case of Balb/c to ca. 2.5 months in the case of Balb/cfC3H (Figure 1). Once tumors begin to appear however, onset rate is approximately the same in the two models (Figure 1). The presence of infectious virus, therefore, facilitates the accumulation of lesions prior to, and which culminate in neoplastic growth.

Hyperplastic alveolar nodules (HAN) begin to be detectable before alveolar adenocarcinomas begin to appear in both the hormone- and virus-predominant models [2,12]. Cells in HAN are pretumorous and the pretumorous condition of cells in HAN is irreversible with respect

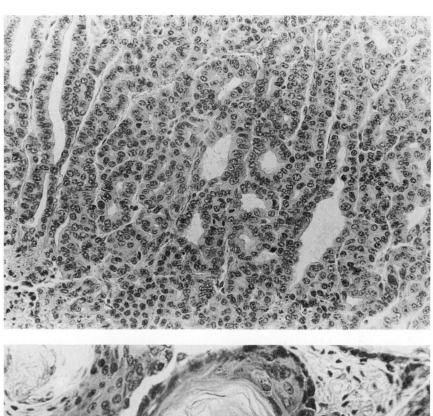

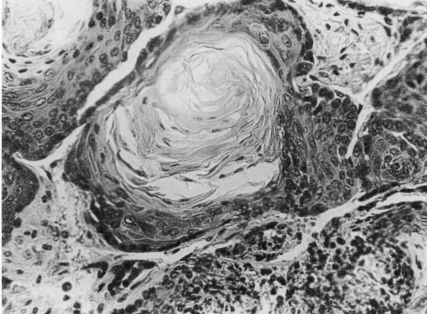

Figure 2. Photomicrographs of illustrative sections of Primary Mammary tumors arising in HI-treated Balb/c mice. A. Primary adeno-carcinoma induced after 13 months of HI treatment. B. Primary adenoacanthoma (showing squamous metaplasia) which developed after 10 months of HI stimulation.

to the hormonal perturbation involved in HAN formation [12]. The
effect of MuMTV-S in enhancing the rate of carcinoma development in
Balb/cfC3H appears to be due primarily to enhancing the rate of HAN
onset. This interpretation is based on our observation that when the
time difference in HAN onset observed in Balb/c and Balb/cfC3H females
is normalized, which is accomplished by isolating and transplanting
HAN into virgin Balb/c females, essentially the same spectrum both
in rates of tumor onset and final tumor incidence are observed for
Balb/cfC3H as for Balb/c HAN's [5]. The same conclusion emerges from
a comparison of data from two other laboratories in which a series
of hyperplastic outgrowth lines induced in Balb/c's by hypophyseal
transplants had a spectrum of tumorigenicities ranging from ca. 10%
to 80% [12] and a series developed in Balb/cfC3H which showed a nearly
identical spectrum of tumorigenic potentials [13]. This data is consistent with the model of infectious virus action as an early event
in neoplastic transformation put forth by DeOme and his colleagues
some years ago [14].

The Action of HI on Hyperplastic Parenchyma

HI cause a non-cyclic hyperplastic proliferation of mammary parenchyma
as early as one month after HI implantation and until the HI graft
is removed [10,11]. The appearance of adenoacanthomas and carcinomas
in the Balb/c mammary gland is preceded by development of many kinds
of focal atypias in hyperplastic parenchyma. These are characterized
histologically by multi-layering of alveoli (adenosis) and by a thick-
ening of ducts (epitheliosis [11]). The neoplastic potential of all
the various pre-cancerous atypias that develop is not well known.
Not all lesions, however, appear to be truly precancerous. We tested
several focal atypias that developed during the first 14 months of
HI treatment in Balb/c; all were reversible, requiring continued hormonal perturbation (HI) for maintainance. Transplantation of tissue
containing these dysplastic foci, into virgin females, resulted in
only normal ductal outgrowths (Table 1). Whether these reversible
growth responses to carcinogenic hormonal regimens represent early

TABLE 1
Instability of the HI-Induced Hyperplastic Growth Phenotype[a]

No. Months in HI Hosts (Donor)	Implantation (Recipient)	Number Transplants (Recipient)	Number Hyperplastic Outgrowths[b]	Number Tumors
6	F	7	0	0
8	F	4	0	0
10	F	5	0	0
11	F	6	0	0
11	D	8	0	0
12	F	7	0	0
14	F	7	0	0
14	F (HI-3)	4	3	0

[a]One mm^3 fragments (F) of hyperplastic tissue were excised from glands of HI females at the designated length of time after introduction of HI (Donor). Dissociated cells (D) were obtained by collagenase digestion of I hyperplastic gland (see [32] for method). Both fragments and dissociated cells (1 X 10^6) were inoculated into cleared glands of 3 week old virgin recipients and left for a minimum of 3 months (3-10 months). Hyperplasia was measured against an HI-implanted control recipient (HI-3 above, which corresponds to tissue transplanted for 3 months in HI rather than virgin females).
[b]Although no outgrowth exhibited hyperplastic growth potential in virgin females which was comparable to that observed in HI recipients, focal dysplasias, primarily adenosis and peri-ductal fibrosis, did occur in 48% of outgrowth tissues.

changes with a cancerous endpoint or rather represent benign end-point changes unrelated to cancer has not been determined, but is of obvious importance in understanding the significance of early atypical hyperplasia in hormonal carcinogenesis.

HI do facilitate the development of tumors in HAN [12]. In our hands, the effect of HI has been most dramatic in the D2 HAN outgrowth developed by Medina in Balb/c, in the hormone-predominant model [12]. The effect of HI on tumor onset and incidence in the D2 HAN is shown in Figure 3. The hormone treatment decreased tumor latency from 6 months to 2 months and increased final incidence from 27% to 100%. Approximately 70% of these tumors appeared in a two month interval,

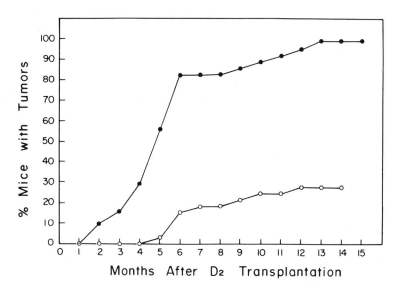

Figure 3. The Effect of HI on Mammary Tumor Development in the D2 Hyperplasia. 3-4 week old mice received 1 mm^3 pieces of the transplanted D2 outgrowth in the cleared fat pad of the #4 mammary gland. The outgrowth was in the 47th transplant generation. Thirty-one mice received 2 hypophyseal isografts under the kidney capsule (●). Thirty-four mice served as controls (O). The mice were palpated monthly for appearance of tumors.

between 3 and 5 months after beginning HI treatment. Because of this dramatic effect of HI, we used the D2 outgrowth in an attempt to define how hormones acted to facilitate tumor onset in the hyperplastic tissue.

We first considered that HI selected latent tumorigenic cells. If HI acted to select covert tumor cells, the tumors should behave in predictable ways; they should be dependent upon or at least responsive to HI for proliferation. Our data is not consistent with that idea. First, tumor cells from HI-induced tumors grew as well in virgin females as did tumor cells from control hosts (Table 2). Second, if HI only acted to enhance the rate of tumor appearance by selecting responsive tumor cells, we would have expected the final tumor incidence in the control group (Figure 3) to approach 100%. However, the tumor incidence in control hosts was only 27%. Therefore, we consider

TABLE 2
Onset of HI-Induced D2 Tumors in Control Virgin Hosts[a]

Tumor Origin		Virgin Recipient	
HI/V	Onset Time (Months)	Incidence	Onset Time (Days)
HI	3	100%	11, 14
HI	4	100%	9, 14
V	9	100%	14, 17
V	10	100%	10, 11

[a]Tumors occurred either in HI or virgin (V) hosts at the indicated time after D2 HAN transplantation. Fragments of tumor approximately $1mm^3$ were inoculated subcutaneously in two virgin recipients and onset time monitored daily thereafter.

that HI did not act simply to select pre-existing tumor cells in increasing tumor incidence and decreasing onset time.

HI did not significantly change the rate at which the D2 hyperplastic tissue grew to fill mammary fat (Figure 4). Therefore, HI did not likely act to induce carcinomas through an indirect effect of increasing proliferation rate of hyperplastic cells. There was, nonetheless, with three exceptions, a direct relationship between growth rate of a given hyperplastic outgrowth and the occurrence of a tumor in it, that was, however, not related to HI treatment (Figure 5).

A minimum of 2 months HI treatment was required for the maximum tumorigenic response of D2 pretumorous cells (Figure 6). Treatment for one month resulted in tumors at approximately the same frequency as in virgin controls. Thus, the effect of HI could be reversed if removed sufficiently early in the evolution of tumors. Likewise, the two month HI treatment had to be consecutive for maximum effectiveness. If the two treatment months were interrupted for one month, the effect was to reduce tumor frequency to below control, virgin values (Figure 6). Thus, the maximum effect of HI in tumor onset appeared also to be non-additive.

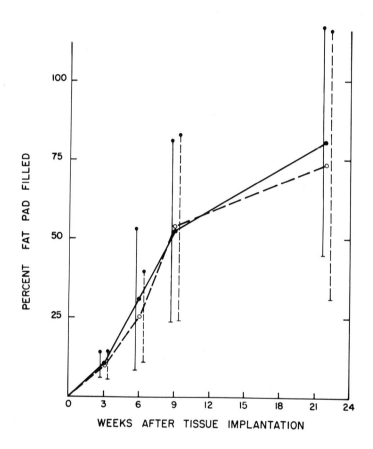

Figure 4. Effect of HI on Growth of the D2 Hyperplasia. One mm³ fragment of the D2 hyperplastic outgrowth was implanted into the cleared Balb/c mammary glands of 80 3-4 week old female mice. Half received 3 HI under their kidney capsules (●). The other half served as controls (O). The extent of outgrowth was measured in each animal at 4 consecutive times (3,6,9 and 21 weeks after tissue implantation). Thus, growth curves were established for each outgrowth fragment in each animal. The mean and standard error for all growth curves is shown. Growth was measured as a linear percent of the cleared fat pad occupied, using vernier calipers.

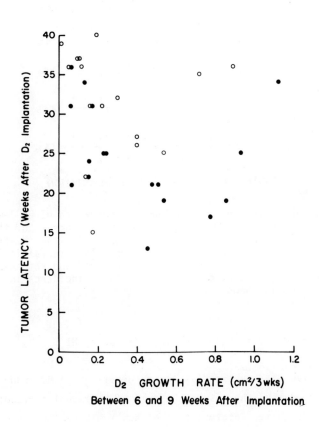

Figure 5. Relationship Between Growth Rate and Tumor Onset Time in the D2 Hyperplastic Outgrowths. The growth rate of 16 individual D2 hyperplastic outgrowths in HI hosts and 16 outgrowths in control hosts, described in the legend to Figure 4, each of which formed tumors, is plotted against the onset time for the development of the tumor within it (tumor latency). In this case, the area of outgrowth was used as the growth parameter. The result was the same if percent fat pad filled was used instead. Growth rate during time of maximum outgrowth (between 6 and 9 weeks; see Figure 4) is shown. Solid symbols, HI treated; open symbols, control tissue.

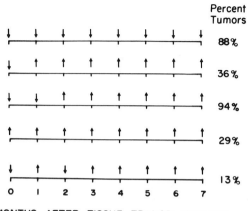

Percent
Tumors

88%

36%

94%

29%

13%

0   1   2   3   4   5   6   7

MONTHS AFTER TISSUE TRANSPLANTATION

Figure 6. The Effect of Discontinuous Exposure to HI on Tumor Formation in D2 Hyperplastic Outgrowths. One mm^3 fragments of the D2 hyperplasia were introduced into cleared fat pads of either HI-treated (↓)
or control (↑) Balb/c females. At the monthly interval indicated
thereafter, similar size fragments were removed and retransplanted
either in HI (↓) or control (↑) hosts. Tumor incidence in 21-30 animals per group is shown.

Induction of MuMTV in Balb/c Mammary Tissue by HI

The objective of these studies was to determine if HI induced MuMTV
at any time during the natural history of "hormonal carcinogenesis".
This study required determination of how MuMTV was expressed in normal
mammary glands of Balb/c females during physiologic hormonal stimulation of pregnancy. Details of these studies have recently been presented elsewhere [11]. We therefore, in what follows, point out only
the major finding.

We first established that the Balb/c colony used for these studies
contained only endogenous MuMTV provirus-sequences in mammary gland
DNA. We then determined how MuMTV was expressed in mammary parenchyma.

In a survey of mammary glands from over 199 first-pregnant females, MuMTV core (p28) or envelope (gp52) antigens were not detected
in immunoperoxidase assays using MuMTV-S sera, or in interspecies

radioimmunassays. The sensitivity of these methods suggested that less than one cell in 1,000 or less than one ng/mg normal cell protein was sufficiently related to the major structural proteins of MuMTV for detection. Essentially identical results were obtained whether glands of young (3-6 months) or older (9 and 12 month) pregnant females were used (Table 3). Mammary cells of mice in first pregnancy also contained very low concentrations of MuMTV-S related RNA sequences, corresponding to an average of less than 0.1 equivalent (0.0001% ± 0.00004%) of MuMTV 35S RNA per cell (Table 3).

HI did not induce expression of either RNA or structural antigens in mammary tissue during its hyperplasiogenic effect on that tissue (Table 3). Genomic RNA remained at less than 0.1 equivalent per cell in non-tumor glands, tested monthly during a 14 month course of HI treatment [11].

MuMTV structural antigens were detected in cells of HI-induced primary mammary tumors. MuMTV p28 was detected in each of 4 tumors tested by interspecies RIA (Table 3). Gp52 was detected in 1 of 4 tumors tested in interspecies radioimmunoassays (Table 3). In immunoperoxidase assays, 5 of 8 tumors tested contained gp52-reactive cells, though these cells were quite infrequent in tissue samples [11].

RNA from HI-induced tumors contained between 1 and 600 equivalents of MuMTV 355 RNA (average) per cell (Table 3). The increased MuMTV RNA content in tumors was not, however, dependent on HI once the tumors were formed; the same concentration was detected in each of two tumors transplanted in virgin hosts as was detected in the primary tumors in HI-containing hosts (data not shown).

Two alveolar hyperplasias (PH-1 [15] and D2 [12]) also contained elevated amounts of MuMTV-related markers (Table 3). PH-1 tissue contained areas where a high percentage (60-95%) p28-reactive cells were observed as well as areas in which no cells were reactive. D2 contained areas in which as many as 45% cells were reactive, as well as entirely negative areas (Table 3). Gp52 was not detected in either hyperplasia (Table 3). Multiple equivalents of an MuMTV-S-related genome were detected in both hyperplasias (Table 3).

TABLE 3
Summary of MuMTV Expression in HI-Induced Neoplasms

Tissue[a]	HI	Immunoreactive Protein (ng/mg)[b]		Percent Cells Reactive With[c]		RNA[d]	
		p28	gp52	Anti-gp52	Anti-p28	Genome Equivalent/Cell	(+1°C)
Normal	+	<1.0	<1.0	<0.1	<0.1	<0.1[e]	82
Dysplastic	+	<1.0	<1.0	<0.1	<0.1	<0.1	81
Control	-	<1.0	<1.0	<0.1	<0.1	<0.1	82
D2 HAN	-	ND[g]	ND	<0.1	6-34	4400±316	80
D2 HAN	+	ND	ND	<0.1	2-35	1850±216	81
PH-1 HAN	-	ND	ND	<0.1	70-95	1100±360	81
Primary tumor[f]	+	8-2000	1-880	<0.1-35	<0.1-95	1-600	81-83
PH-1 tumor	-	ND	ND	1-3	60-95	400±66	83
D2 tumor	-	ND	ND	1-7	33-45	360±44	83
Balb/cfC3H tumor	-	2600	1000	35-70	90-95	3300	88

aNormal tissue = glands of HI-treated females with no evidence of adenosis or epitheliosis 1,3 and 6 months after HI treatment. Dysplastic = tissue from HI treated females with focal adenosis or epitheliosis 6,9 and 12 months after HI treatment. Control tissues are mammary tissues from first mid to late pregnant females, age matched with HI-treated females. D2 and PH-1 are premalignant alveolar hyperplasias with tumor incidences of 33% and 30% respectively, in virgin Balb/c female hosts. HI treatment in D2 bearing hosts was from 2 to 6 months.

bResults of interspecies radioimmunoassays conducted by Y. Teramoto and J. Schlom (see 31).

cResults of immunoperoxidase assays using MuMTV-S antisera (see 11 for methodologic detail); Maxima and minima (above background of 0.1) for a minimum of 10 positive random microscopic fields (X250) are shown. Unreactive areas were also present in all reactive tissues.

dData are from determinations on a minimum of 2 (2-5) tissue samples. MuMTV-S cDNA$_{rep}$ was used in hybridizations and thermal denaturations described in (11).

eThe 0.1 value was obtained by extrapolating from hybridization rate curves which did not approach 50% cDNA hybridization (11). Tms were determined on RNA selected from these tissues by affinity chromatography on Oligo dT. This pre-selection enriched for MuMTV-related sequences approximately 100-fold (11).

fData are from tumors with 0-40% approximate fractional area of squamous metaplasia, determined from 1-2 histologic sections. Age of first tumor palpability is from 8-21 months. Maxima and minima for each assay is shown; RIA, immunoperoxidase and RNA assays were performed on 4, 8 and 5 individual tumors, respectively.

gND = Not determined. These data can be found in reference 31 and confirm non-coordinate suppression of gp52 seen in immunoperoxidase data.

The tumors derived from both hyperplasias contained areas of high
(95%) and low (<0.1%) p28 reactivity [11]. Gp52 was detected in a
small but significant fraction (1-7% maximum) in tumors derived from
both hyperplasias [11].

HI stimulation did not change the expression of MuMTV p28, gp52
or RNA in the D2 hyperplasia (Table 3). The number of p28-reactive
cells did increase from a maximum of less than 10% to a maximum of
about 35% during the time from month 2 to month 4 after HI, but the
increase in p28-reactive cells from month 2 to month 4 was approximately the same in control tissue ([11], Table 3). Gp52 was not detected
in immunoperoxidase assays (using MuMTV-S antisera) at either 2, 4
or 6 months after transplantation (Table 3) in either control or HI
hosts.

In HI hosts, MuMTV RNA concentrations in D2 hyperplasias were
even less (about 2.5 fold) than in control hosts. This difference
was not likely due to the presence of different amounts of hyperplastic
tissue, since outgrowth size increased at approximately the same rate
in HI as in control hosts (Figure 4).

HI also did not increase the number of p28 or gp52 reactive cells
or RNA levels in D2 tumors over that observed in control hosts (data
not shown).

The MuMTV Expressed in HI-Induced Neoplastic Balb/c Tissues is Replication-Defective

B-type particles have not been detected, either budding or mature,
in samples of PH-1 or D2 hyperplasias, or D2 tumors (Table 4). As
observed in tissue sections, expression of p28 and gp52 in cells in
primary cultures of PH-1 and D2 hyperplasias was non-coordinate, where
gp52 was not detected and p28 was detected in a major fraction of cells
with MuMTV-S sera (Table 4). No particles containing MuMTV-related
RNA could be detected in supernatant media of these cultures. We
therefore conclude that the MuMTV expressed in Balb/c pretumorous
hyperplasia, called MuMTV (HIN-B) is replication defective. The RNA
of this virus-like RNA in premalignant Balb/c tissues was readily

TABLE 4
Defectiveness of MuMTV (HIN-B)

	Tumor Cells	Culture Cells		Culture Field
	No Positive for B Particles[a]	% Reactive[b] gp52	p28	% Hybridization at Crt = 10[c]
PH-1	0/70	0	790	0
PH-1 tumor	NT	0	80-90	0
D-2	0/1200	0	35-60	NT
D-2 tumor	0/100	0	60-80	0
Balb/cfC3H tumor	18/35	60-85	790	100

[a]Transmission electron microscopic data on duplicate tissue samples in which the total number of cells screened (and positive) is shown. D2 tissues were in HI-stimulated hosts, PH-1 tissues were in virgin hosts. NT is not tested.
[b]Immunofluorescence data on triplicate acetone-fixed cultures.
[c]Supernatant medium (48 hr.) from confluent cultures was clarified by 800xg centrifugation. RNA was purified from 100,000xg pellets of the supernatant as described in Methods. RNA was hybridized in duplicate to MuMTV cDNA$_{rep}$.

distinguishable from MuMTV-S RNA by a 6-8°C lower Tm of hybrids (Table 3; [11]) formed with MuMTV-S cDNA. In fact, the Tm of hybrids formed between RNA from all the Balb/c neoplasms we tested and MuMTV-S cDNA was 6-8°C lower than RNA from Balb/cfC3H tumors with the same cDNA (Table 3).

DISCUSSION

The purpose of these investigations was to determine if HI, acting to facilitate tumor onset in Balb/c females, induced MuMTV structural information enroute. Because of the large number and variable histories of Balb/c colonies used by different investigators in similar kinds of studies [16], it is necessary to define the natural history of hormonal carcinogenesis carefully in order to compare with data

obtained from these studies. Much of the natural history data on mammary cancer in Balb/c and Balb/cfC3H females in response to HI have
been presented and interpreted in other contexts elsewhere [2,5,11].
Here, we will deal with two concepts not considered in those publications, the evidence that hormones act as mammary tumor promoters and
the possible involvement of replication-defective viruses in hormonal
mammary carcinogenesis in Balb/c mice.

Hormones as Mammary Tumor Promoters

Weinstein et al. summarized the biologic properties of known tumor
promoters [17]. These are shown in Table 5. To this list we have
added the property of hyperplasiogenesis since all known tumor promoters also induce epithelial hyperplasia [18]. We have compared the
action of the hormonal perturbation induced by hypophyseal isografts
(HI) in the formation of mammary tumors in Balb/c to these actions
of known tumor promoters to determine if they might be analogous. A
comparison of their properties suggest that HI and tumor promoters
do act in some analogous ways. HI certainly induced hyperplasia of
mammary epithelium (Figure 2; [11]). Its effect on tumor onset in
the D2 alveolar hyperplasia was also reversible, at least in early
stages of tumor formation. The effect of HI in tumor formation in
the D2 hyperplasia was also non-additive since two treatments of 1
month duration each which was interrupted by one month, was not as
effective as one continuous two month treatment. Indeed the interrupted treatment was actually less effective in tumor onset than no treatment at all. Prolonged treatment was also required in the context of
tumor onset time.

Despite these similarities in biologic action between HI and
known tumor promoters, other comparisons between them cannot be made.
Although direct treatments with some hormones will cause mammary cancer, there are likely many steps at which those hormones might act
in the natural history of disease onset, and no direct hormonal in-
ducer of tumors in hyperplastic tissue has been identified. Indeed,
it may be a particular balance of hormones that is important in

TABLE 5
Biologic Properties of Promoting Agents

1. Hyperplasiogenic

2. Action is reversible (at early stage)

3. Action is not additive

4. Require prolonged exposure

5. No evidence of covalent binding

6. Not mutagenic

7. Not carcinogenic alone

8. Must be given after the initiating agent

9. Probable threshold dose-response

Source: Adapted from [17] and [18].

influencing mammary cancer onset in hyperplasias, rather than any particular hormone effector [19]. Nonetheless, hormones which have been implicated circumstantially in tumor onset (prolactin, progesterone and estrogens) do not, as biologically active hormone-receptor complexes, bind effector molecules covalently [20], nor have they demonstrated mutagenicity [21]. Thus, the available data regarding hormones in mammary tumor onset can be organized into a strong, but circumstantial argument for promotion. Proof for this idea awaits more studies with defined hormone effectors using cells cloned from hyperplastic, premalignant tissues.

Indeed, the action of hormones as mammary tumor promoters begs the existence of initiated cells in pretumorous hyperplasias. Such non-tumorigenic cells, with genetic lesions, at higher than normal risk to form tumors, have not been identified or isolated. Without the isolation of such cells, the argument that hormones act to enhance tumor development in hyperplastic tissue by selecting pre-existing tumor cells [22] must be considered. In the present experiments, we did not detect HI-responsive tumors developed in D2 hyperplasias,

which we would have anticipated if HI simply selected pre-existing
tumor cells from the tissue. Our result, while indirect evidence,
is therefore most consistent with the presence of initiated cells.
It is nonetheless still possible that HI acted to select tumorigenic
cells in the D2 hyperplasia by some indirect effect on an HI-sensitive
arm of a multicomponent biologic unit which acted in the absence of
HI to keep putative tumorigenic cells in check [22].

Mediation of Hormonal Carcinogenesis in Balb/c by Replication-Defective MuMTV

Was the action of HI in mammary tumor onset mediated by its induction
of viral information? Finding induced MuMTV markers in each of 10
primary tumors tested [11] and both of 2 premalignant hyperplasias
and their derivative tumors suggest that possibility circumstantially.
Other investigators have reported similar findings in hormone-induced
neoplasms [22,23]; others have failed to detect MuMTV markers in primary Balb/c mammary tumors of unknown etiology [24-27]. A number of
reconciling explanations, among them different contents of metaplastic
squamous tissue non-supportive of MuMTV replication in tumors, age
of animals at tumor onset, accidental infection with MuMTV, and different effects of different carcinogens on cells, have recently been
discussed [11].

The MuMTV-variant we observed in our studies of hormone-induced
mammary neoplasm was replication-defective. In this property, HIN-B
is different from MTV-O, isolated from aged tumor-bearing mice by
Bentvelzen and his colleagues (see [1] and [11]). In its defectiveness, and also in its genetic distinctiveness from MuMTV-S, HIN-B is
also different from the MuMTV variant(s) expressed in Balb/c mammary
epithelium after MuMTV-S infection (Balb/cfC3H tumors). Varmus et al.
[22] earlier noted a similar distinctiveness of MuMTV-related RNA in
Balb/c mammary neoplasms of unknown etiology and tentatively attributed
the difference to MuMTV strain differences.

All known acutely transforming murine and avian leukemia viruses
and sarcoma viruses are replication-defective, and their transforming
property is related to the recombinations with cell genes that render
them defective [28]. The MCF and related viruses, which are recombinants in the envelope gene between xenotropic, endogenous and ectropic
MuLVs [29,30] may be especially relevant to the present study. Recombinations in the envelope gene made the product of that gene undetectable in MCF viruses, even in interspecies assays with most available
sera [30]. Our inability to detect gp52 related to MuMTV in intraspecies immunoperoxidase assays and interspecies radioimmunoassays
[31] may be due to a similar phenomenon in hormone-induced Balb/c neoplasms. That possibility is under study.

The ubiquity of induced MuMTV footprints in HI-induced neoplasms
and the precedent provided by replication-defective C-type viruses
in cell transformation can be collected into a circumstantial case
for involvement of MuMTV in hormonal carcinogenesis of Balb/c mammary
epithelium. The hormonal perturbation that caused mammary tumors did
not, however, itself induce the defective MuMTV variant. This suggests
that even if HIN-B or related viruses were involved in tumor onset,
some change other than presentation of the hormonal perturbation was
necessary for the virus information to be activated and effective.
The failure of HI to induce MuMTV in normal cells in vivo is consistent
with our inability to induce MuMTV in normal cells in vitro with gluco-
corticoids that led to the notion that an earlier lesion is important
in carcinogenesis that renders the cell susceptible to the virus activating influence of hormones [5]. The nature of the earlier change
that is required for virus activation by hormones is entirely specula-
tive and may be either viral or non-viral. We have suggestive evidence, based on experiments with BudR, that the change is in DNA [5].

Michalides et al. [16] reported that HI did induce MuMTV RNA
structural polypeptides in Balb/c mammary glands. These data are difficult to reconcile with ours, but probably represent differences in
the two Balb/c colonies studied. One reconciling interpretation would

be that the events necessary to sensitize mammary cells to the MuMTV-inductive effect of HI have already occurred in the Balb/c colony used in the study of Michalides et al. [16].

REFERENCES

1. Bentvelzen, P., *Biochem. Biophys. Acta., 355*:236-289 (1974).

2. Nandi, S., and McGrath, C. M., *Advances Cancer Res., 17*:353-414 (1973).

3. Heston, W. E., and Vlahakis, W. E., *J. Natl. Cancer Inst., 40*: 1161-1166 (1968).

4. Morris, V. L., Medeiros, E., Ringold, G. M., Bishop, J. M., and Varmus, H. E., *J. Mol. Biol., 114*:73-91 (1977).

5. McGrath, C. M., and Jones, R. F., *Cancer Res., 38*:4112-4125 (1978).

6. Bern, H., and Nandi, S., *Proc. Exptl. Tumor Res., 2*:90-144 (1961).

7. Muhlbock, O., In: Adv. Cancer Res. IV (J. P. Greenstein, A. Haddow, eds.), Academic Press, New York, 1956, pp. 371-391.

8. Shimkin, M. B., In: Mammary tumors in mice (F. R. Moulton, ed.), AAAS Press, Washington, D.C., 1945, pp. 85-122.

9. Loeb, L., and Kirtz, M. M., *Am. J. Cancer, 36*:56-82 (1939).

10. Muhlbock, O., and Boot, L. M., *Cancer Res., 19*:402-412 (1959).

11. McGrath, C. M., Prass, W. A., Maloney, T. M., and Jones, R. F., *J. Natl. Cancer Inst.,* in press (1981).

12. Medina, D., *Methods Cancer Res., 7*:3-53 (1973).

13. Ashley, R. L., Cardiff, R. D., Mitchell, D. J., Faulkin, L. J., and Lund, J. K., *Cancer Res., 40*:4232 (1980).

14. DeOme, K. B., and Medina, D., *Cancer, 24*:1255 (1969).

15. McGrath, C. M., Marineau, E. J., and Voyles, B. A., *Virology, 87*:339-353 (1978).

16. Michalides, R., VanDeemter, L., Nusse, R., and Hageman, J., *Virology, 31*:63-72 (1979).

17. Weinstein, I. B., Wigler, M., Fisher, P. B., Sisskin, E., and Pietropaolo C., In: Carcinogenesis--A Comprehensive Survey, Vol. 2, Mechanisms of Tumor Promotion and Cocarcinogenesis (T. Slaga, A. Sivak, and R. K. Boutwell, eds.), Raven Press, New York, 1978, pp. 313-334.

18. Marks, F., Bertsch, S., Grimm, W., and Schweizer, J., In: Carcinogenesis--A Comprehensive Survey, Vol. 2, Mechanisms of Tumor Promotion and Cocarcinogenesis (T. Slaga, A. Sivak, and R. K. Boutwell, eds.), Raven Press, New York, 1978, pp. 97-116.

19. Dorenman, S. G., *Cancer, 46*:874-878 (1980).

20. Maurer, H. R., and Chalkley, G. R., *J. Mol. Biol., 27*:431-441 (1967).

21. Nandi, S., *Cancer Res., 38*:4046-4049 (1978).

22. DeOme, K. B., Miyamoto, M. J., Osborn, R. C., Guzman, R. C., and Lum, K., *Cancer Res., 38*:2103-2111 (1978).

23. Varmus, H. E., Quinbrell, N., Medeiros, E., Bishop, J. M., Nowinski, C., and Sarkar, N. H., *J. Mol. Biol., 79*:663-679 (1973).

24. Moore, D. H., Sarkar, N. H., Holben, J. A., and Sheffield, J. B., *Int. J. Cancer, 23*:713-717 (1979).

25. Schlom, J., Michalides, R., Kufe, D., Hehlmann, R., Spiegelman, S., Bentvelzen, P., and Hageman, P., *J. Natl. Cancer Inst., 51*:541-551 (1973).

26. Pauley, R. J., Medina, D., and Socher, S. H., *J. Virol., 29*:483-493 (1979).

27. Pauley, R. J., Medina, D., and Socher, S. H., *J. Virol., 32*:557-566 (1979).

28. Aaronson, S. A., and Stephenson, J. R., *Biochem. Biophys. Acta., 458*:323-354 (1976).

29. Elder, J. H., Gautsch, J. W., Jensen, F. C., Lerner, R. A., Hartley, J. W., and Rowe, W. P., *Proc. Natl. Acad. Sci., U.S.A., 74*:4676-4681 (1977).

30. Ruscetti, S., Linemeyer, D., Feild, J., Troxler, D., and Scolnick, E., *J. Exp. Med., 148*:654-663 (1978).

31. Teramoto, Y. A., Medina, D., McGrath, C. and Schlom, J., *Virology,* 345-353 (1980).

32. Voyles, B. A., and McGrath, C. M., *Int. J. Cancer, 18*:498-509 (1976).

SEPARATE PATHWAYS FOR VIRAL AND CHEMICAL CARCINOGENESIS
IN THE MOUSE MAMMARY GLAND

Larry O. Arthur

Biological Carcinogenesis Program
Frederick Cancer Research Center
Frederick, Maryland

Janet S. Butel

Departmnet of Virology
Baylor College of Medicine
Houston, Texas

Daniel Medina
Sandra K. Dusing-Swartz
Susan H. Socher

Department of Cell Biology
Baylor College of Medicine
Houston, Texas

Gilbert H. Smith

Laboratory of Molecular Biology
National Cancer Institute
Bethesda, Maryland

INTRODUCTION

Since 1946, a number of investigators have demonstrated that chemical carcinogens induce mammary tumors in a variety of mouse strains with and without exogenous MMTV [1-14]. In most studies, a 40-70% incidence by 10-14 months occurs in virgin mice treated with either 3-methylcholanthrene (MCA), 7,12-dimethylbenzanthracene (DMBA), or urethane. By 10 months, a significant incidence of leukemias, stomach tumors, ovarian tumors, and lung tumors arise, so many experiments do not progress beyond 12 months of host age.

The induction of mammary tumors by chemical carcinogens has been formulated into two general hypotheses. One hypothesis considers that the two carcinogens act on separate target cells which leads to separate developmental pathways [12,13,15]. This hypothesis emphasizes

169

the differences in cellular origin of mammary cancer and secondarily considers the molecular origin. The second hypothesis, proposed originally by Peter Bentvelzen and co-workers [7,10,14], considers that chemical carcinogens activate an endogenous MMTV which is the ultimate carcinogen. A corollary to this latter hypothesis would suggest that both exogenous MMTV and chemical carcinogens act on a common host cell site altering expression of a regulatory protein. This hypothesis attempts to unify chemical and viral mechanisms of action and does not address the cellular origin of mammary cancer.

As originally formulated, the two hypotheses address different aspects of chemical carcinogen-induced mammary tumors and thus, they are not mutually exclusive. In addressing these two questions, we have investigated the interaction of chemical carcinogens with exogenous and endogenous MMTV in several different mouse systems, with the ultimate goal of determining the extent and mechanism of interaction between the two types of oncogens.

Evidence for Separate Developmental Pathways

The first evidence that chemical carcinogen-induced mammary tumors might evolve differently than viral-induced mammary tumors came from studies on the morphological precursors to the mammary tumors [11,13, 15,16]. Table 1 illustrates the incidence of mammary dysplasias in C3H/StWi virgin mice. Mice infected with MMTV give rise primarily to alveolar hyperplasias (HAN), whereas the same mice treated with chemical carcinogens contain primarily ductal hyperplasias (DH) [16, 17]. Mice infected with MMTV and treated with DMBA contain both types of hyperplasias [17]. These same results were obtained also in BALB/c

TABLE 1
Induction of Mammary Dysplasias in Virgin C3H/StWi Mice

Agent	No. Mice with HAN Total Mice	(%)	$\overline{X}$ HAN Positive Mouse	No. Mice with DH Total Mice	(%)	$\overline{X}$ DH Positive Mouse
MMTV[a]	13/15	(87)	25.0	0/15	(0)	---
DMBA (6 mg)	0/15	(0)	----	11/15	(73)	3.6

[a]C3H/StWi mice were foster-nursed on C3H/He to introduce MMTV-S. The mice were subsequently brother X sister mated to establish an MMTV-S infected C3H/St substrain [16].

and C57BL mice [11,13,15]. It appears DH are more frequent lesions
than alveolar hyperplasias in chemical carcinogen-treated mice. The
data suggest that in virgin mice, mammary tumors can evolve along
different cellular pathways depending on the etiological agents.
However, chemical carcinogen treatment of the hormonally stimulated
mammary gland (where alveolar differentiation is extensive) induces
both ductal and alveolar hyperplasias, the latter exhibiting a marked
degree of squamous metaplasia [13,15,18]. Chemical carcinogen induction of alveolar hyperplasias can be recapitulated in vitro. Banerjee
and co-workers [19,20] have demonstrated that DMBA, and not noncarcinogenic analogs, induces nodule-like alveolar lesions in organ culture
provided the mammary tissue exhibits alveolar differentiation. Upon
transplantation these alveolar lesions produce alveolar hyperplasias
morphologically similar to viral induced alveolar hyperplasias, and
give rise to mammary tumors [20]. Thus, within the same mouse strain,
it appears DMBA and other chemical carcinogens can give rise to ductal
and alveolar hyperplasias, depending on the differentiative state of
the mammary gland. Our working hypothesis emphasizes that viral and
chemical carcinogens transform different target cells in the virgin
mouse. Exogenous MMTV may transform the alveolar cell or alveolar
stem cell whereas DMBA may transform the ductal cell or ductal stem
cell. In the hormonally stimulated mammary gland, DMBA transforms
both alveolar and ductal cells. It is important to emphasize that
the existence of different stem cell compartments has only been in-
ferred and not experimentally demonstrated for the mammary gland.

Evidence of the Activation of Endogenous Virus

Given that the 2 carcinogens yield different morphological precursors
in the virgin mouse, what is the evidence that the chemical carcinogens
may be activating an endogenous MMTV?

Bentvelzen and co-workers [9,10,14] provided evidence that MMTV
antigens could be demonstrated in the spleens of irradiated or urethane
urethane-treated C57BL mice; irradiation/urethane leads to production
of virions in 020 mice; and in aged BALB/c mice, mature virions are

TABLE 2
MMTV RNA Levels in DMBA-Induced Mammary Tumors

Strain	Mice with Tumors / Total Mice	(%)	MMTV RNA (% of Total RNA)		Range MMTV RNA
C3H/StWi	17/37	(46)	0.0023	(5)[a]	(0.005-0.0044)
C3H/StWi controls[b]	0/62	(0)	0.0035	(1)	--
BD2F$_1$	24/35	(69)	0.007	(4)	(0.001-0.019)
BD2F$_1$ controls[c]	0/43	(0)	0.006	(4)	(0.002-0.011)

[a] Number in parentheses, number of samples.
[b] Pooled mammary glands from 5 retired breeders.
[c] 12-month-old untreated virgin mice.

expressed in mammary tissues. Michalides, in Holland [21,22], and we have reinvestigated this problem using molecular hybridization and immunocytochemical techniques to detect MMTV expression in mammary tissues of hormone-treated or chemical carcinogen-treated mice. Table 2 shows MMTV RNA levels in 2 mouse strains free of exogenous MMTV, C3H/StWi and BD2F$_1$ [16,23]. DMBA induced 46 and 69% mammary tumor incidence in the two strains, respectively. However, in mammary tumors of both strains, the level of MMTV-specific RNA as detected by molecular hybridization analysis was the same as in normal glandular tissues. The extent of hybridization is shown in Figure 1. In these analyses, hybridization was carried out in RNA excess with a cDNA probe made against MMTV RNA purified from virions produced from Mm5mt cells [24]. The extent of hybridization is plotted as a function of the ratio of input RNA/input cDNA. When purified 70S MMTV RNA is hybridized to the MMTV cDNA probe at low RNA/DNA ratios maximum hybridization (95%) is achieved, whereas tumors from BD2F$_1$ mice show only limited hybridization (40-50%) at high RNA/cDNA ratios (35,000/1). RNA from MMTV-S positive tumors exhibit >80% maximum hybridization at low levels of input RNA under the same conditions [24].

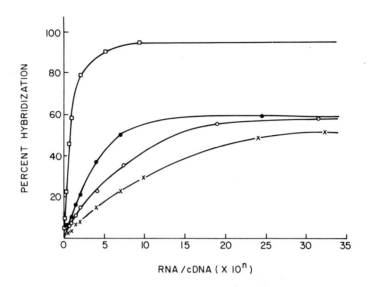

Figure 1. Molecular hybridization of MuMTV cDNA to MuMTV RNA and to total cellular RNA from $BD2F_1$ mammary tissues. The ^3H-labeled MuMTV cDNA was hybridized to increasing amounts of purified 70S MuMTV RNA or to total cellular RNA from mammary tissues as described in [23]. The percentage of hybridization, expressed as a percentage of the input cDNA, is plotted as a function of the ration of input RNA to input cDNA. Hybridization were carried out with 70S MuMTV RNA (□) and with cellular RNA extracted from a $BD2F_1$ mammary gland with 0.011% MuMTV RNA (o), and a DMBA-induced mammary tumor with 0.019% MuMTV RNA (•), and a DMBA induced tumor in an animal bearing a pituitary isograft with 0.007% MuMTV RNA (x). The RNA/cDNA ratios used in these hybridizations were (x 10^0) with 70S MuMTV RNA and (x 10^3) with $BD2F_1$ mammary tissues. (With permission from Cancer Research 40:363-373, 1980).

BALB/c mice have been analyzed more extensively than either C3H or $BD2F_1$, since they have undetectable or very low levels of MMTV RNA ($\leq$ 0.0005% MMTV RNA = 1 MMTV genome equivalent per haploid level of DNA in normal mammary gland tissues). Table 3 shows the expression of MMTV in BALB/c mammary tumors induced by different doses of DMBA alone or in combination with hormonal stimulation. The following results are illustrated in this table. 1) Mammary tumor incidence is similar (25-35%) with 2-6 mg DMBA; however the latent period is inversely correlated with the total dose of DMBA. As the total dose

TABLE 3
Expression of MMTV in Mammary Tumors
Induced in BALB/c Mice by DMBA

Dose of DMBA (mg)	Pituitary Isograft	Tumor Incidence	No. of Tumors with MMTV RNA[a]		
			$\leq$0.0005%	0.006-0.0010%	$\geq$0.0011%
6	No	30[b]	12(75)[c]	4(25)	0(0)
2-4	No	25-35[b]	9(45)	4(20)	7(35)
6	Yes[d]	76	7(88)	1(12)	0(0)
6	Yes[e]	42	3(36)	4(36)	3(27)

[a]MMTV RNA levels calculated as the percent of total cellular RNA.
[b]Mean time of tumor appearance (months after the initial administration of DMBA = 5.5 for 6 mg, 7.2 for 4 mg group, and 9.6 for 2 mg group.
[c]Numbers in parentheses represent percent of tumors in that group.
[d]Pituitary grafted at 4 weeks of host age.
[e]Pituitary grafted at 14 weeks of age.

of DMBA increased, the mean latent period for tumor formation decreased from 9.6 to 5.5 months. 2) As the total dose decreased, more tumors arose which had increased levels of MMTV RNA. In tumors induced by 2-4 mg DMBA, 35% had significantly increased levels of MMTV RNA ($\geq$ 0.0011%), whereas none of the tumors induced by 6 mg DMBA contained these levels. 3) Although hormonal stimulation increased the tumor incidence to 76%, it did not increase the number of tumors with increased levels of MMTV RNA. The mean latent period of tumor formation was 3.5 months. However, if the mice received the pituitary isograft after DMBA was administered, the tumor incidence was only 42%, but some tumors developed with increased levels of MMTV RNA expression. These results suggested that MMTV RNA expression might be correlated with the tumor latency period. Table 4 shows the relationship between tumor latency period and MMTV expression in mammary adenocarcinomas. Only mammary adenocarcinomas were evaluated since they appeared randomly over the time period of the experiment, whereas the vast majority of adenocanthomas appeared by 30 weeks [11,23]. In our experiments, adenocanthomas were defined according to their degree of squamous

TABLE 4

Relationship Between Tumor Latency and MMTV Expression in
Mammary Adenocarcinomas Induced in BALB/c Mice by DMBA

Tumor Latency Period (Weeks)	Total Tumors	No. Tumors with MMTV RNA[a]		
		<0.0005%	0.006-0.0010%	>0.0011%
<30	23	15(65)[b]	4(17)	4(17)
>30	18	8(44)	4(22)	6(33)

[a]MMTV RNA levels expressed as percent of total cellular RNA.
[b]Numbers in parenthesis represent percent of tumors in that group.

metaplasia and keratinization. Any tumor where 25% or more of the
cells exhibited evidence of keratinization at the light microscope
level was considered an adenoacanthoma.

The majority of tumors (65%) appearing before 30 weeks exhibited
undetectable levels of MMTV RNA whereas the majority of tumors (56%)
arising after 30 weeks had increased levels of MMTV RNA, albeit the
mean levels were low (0.0038%; n = 10) compared to tumors arising in
BALB/cfC3H (0.0676%; n = 25). As in C3H/StWi and BD2F$_1$ tumors, the
extent of hybridization was very low; 20% in BALB/c mammary tumors
with detectable levels of MMTV RNA [24]. The results demonstrated
that increased levels of MMTV RNA expression was not correlated with
mammary tumor maintenance and perhaps, not even with tumor induction,
in strains where the MMTV genome was undectable (BALB/c) or only
partially expressed (C3H/StWi, BD2F$_1$).

The next series of experiments examined the effects of DMBA on
the expression of MMTV RNA in mice containing exogenous MMTV. Previous
results had demonstrated that the tumor risk was the same for DMBA-
treated C3H/StWi mice irrespective of the presence or absence of exogenous MMTV-S [17]. In MMTV-S infected mice, untreated with DMBA,
the tumor frequency was low, but measurable. Similar experiments have
been carried out in BALB/cfC3H mice. Although we could not distinguish
between expression of endogenous and exogenous MMTV RNA, the data pro-

TABLE 5
Expression of MMTV in Mammary Tumors Induced
in BALB/cfC3H Mice by DMBA

Dose of DMBA (mg)	Pituitary Isograft	Tumor Incidence	No. Tumors with MMTV RNA[b]		
			≤0.005%	0.0006-0.0010%	>0.0011%
6	No	33	9(25)[c]	3(8)	24(67)
1.5-3.0	No	35-42	10(50)	0(0)	10(50)
6	Yes	100	5(20)	1(4)	19(76)

[a]Mean latent period of tumor formation = 4.6 mo. for 6 mg, 7.0 mo. for 3 mg, 8.6 mo. for 1.5 mg, and 3.3 mo. for 6 mg plus pituitary isograft.
[b]MMTV RNA levels calculated as the percent of total cellular RNA.
[c]Number in parenthesis represents percent of tumors in that group.

vided some unexpected results. Table 5 shows the expression of MMTV in mammary tumors induced in BALB/cfC3H mice by different doses of DMBA. Doses of 1.5 - 6.0 mg DMBA gave a similar tumor incidence of 33-42% but the latency period was inversely proportional to the dose. The interesting observation lay in the appearance of tumors that had undetectable (background) levels of MMTV RNA expression. In virgin mice, 25-50% of the tumors had low levels depending upon the dose of DMBA. When the tumor incidence was high (MMTV-S + pituitary isograft), 20% of the tumors had background levels of MMTV RNA. In mammary adeno-carcinomas induced within the same latent period (10-25 weeks) and with the same dose of DMBA (6 mg), the number of tumors with undetectable levels of RNA was diminished from 41-20% by concomitant hormone stimulation (data not shown). Hormone stimulation either selected for those cells capable of expressing MMTV RNA or stimulated MMTV RNA expression. The latter point has been demonstrated in several MMTV systems [25,27]. The extent of nucleic acid hybridization in these tumors varied from complete to low [24]. These experiments demonstrated no synergism between DMBA and MMTV-S either in tumor induction or MMTV RNA expression.

TABLE 6
Immunoperoxidase Detection of MMTV in DMBA-Induced
Mammary Tumors in BALB/c and BALB/cfC3H Mice

Strain	Immunoperoxidase-Detectable Antigens		
	α-(C3H) MMTV (RC)[a]	α-(C3H) MMTV (LA)[a]	α-(C3Hf) MMTV (LA)
BALB/c[b]	0/16	0/16	0/16
BALB/cfC3H[c]	0/5	0/5	0/5
BALB/cfC3H[b]	8/10	10/10	10/10

[a]Antisera were obtained from Drs. Robert Cardiff (RC) and Larry Arthur (LA).
[b]All tumors were mammary adenocarcinomas with MMTV RNA levels $\geq$ 0.0005%.
[c]All tumors were mammary adenocarcinomas with MMTV RNA levels $\leq$ 0.0005%.

The last series of experiments have examined viral RNA translation in DMBA-induced tumors using immunological methods. The peroxidase-antiperoxidase staining technique was used to examine localization of viral antigens in paraffin sections [23,24,28,29]. Table 6 shows the immunoperoxidase detection of MMTV antigens in DMBA-induced mammary tumors in BALB/c and BALB/cfC3H mice. Three different antisera were used. Two were against purified MMTV virions from the cell line Mm5mt, and the third antisera was against purified virions from a C3Hf mammary tumor cell line [30]. Peroxidase localizations occurred in alveolar lumina and along the apical membranes of tumor cells. In BALB/c tumors whose RNA levels were greater than 0.0005%, none demonstrated reactivity. In contrast, MMTV antigens were detected in BALB/cfC3H with MMTV RNA greater than 0.0005%, but not less than 0.0005%. Table 7 shows the expression of MMTV antigens in DMBA-induced mammary tumors in C3H/StWi and C3H/StMTV mice examined by the peroxidase staining method and by competition radioimmunoassay [30,31]. The antisera used were prepared against purified viral structural proteins, gp52 and p27 [31]. Whereas both antigens were detected in high concentrations and in most cells of the tumors induced in the presence

TABLE 7
Detection of MMTV gp52 and p27 in DMBA-Induced
Mammary Tumors in C3H/StWi and C3H/St MTV Mice

Strain	Immunocytochemical Staining		Competition Radioimmunoassay	
	gp52	p27	gp52	p27
C3H/StWi	1/19[a]	6/19	1/8[b]	2/8[d]
C3H/StMTV	5/5	5/5	7/7[c]	7/7[e]

[a] Numerator = No. of positive tumors; denominator = No. of tumors tested.
[b] 2,900 ug/mg protein.
[c] 23,000 ug/mg protein.
[d] 17,000-22,000 ug/mg protein.
[e] 94,800 ug/mg protein.

of exogenous MMTV (i.e. C3H/StMTV), only a minority of tumors exhibited detectable quantities in those tumors induced in the absence of exogenous MMTV. It appeared that p27 was easier to detect than gp52 in tumors induced in C3H/StWi, however, even in these tumors, the level of antigen was very low compared to C3H/StMTV tumors.

SUMMARY

The available data from 2 different laboratories do not support the general hypothesis that chemical carcinogens activate an endogenous MMTV genome in the induction of murine mammary tumors. Two sets of evidence argue against this hypothesis. First, mammary tumors induced by chemical carcinogens develop through a different cellular pathway than viral induced tumors. The working hypothesis from these results suggest that the 2 different oncogens transform 2 different cell types. A similar hypothesis has been formulated by Slemmer [12] to explain the different mammary tumor types induced by viral and chemical carcinogens. Secondly, the data from numerous experiments demonstrate that chemical carcinogens do not lead to increased MMTV RNA or protein expression in mammary tumors [16,17,21-24]. The biochemical evidence

suggesting that different developmental and perhaps different molecular
pathways exist for the 2 carcinogens. The available data, though com-
pelling, has to be considered within the framework of the available
methodology. So far, the nucleic acid and immunological probes have
been developed against the exogenous virus. While the probes theoreti-
cally recognize all parts of the exogenous viral genome [32], it is
not known whether these probes recognize unique portions of the endogenous MMTV genome or a unique host cell "transforming" gene. It
would be very informative to determine which parts of MMTV genome are
being expressed preferentially in the carcinogen-induced mammary tumor
tumors. Until cloned probes of MMTV are available from MMTV-S, MMTV-L
and other MMTVs which can be used to evaluate the qualitative nature
of the genome which is expressed in these tumors as well as probes
for evaluating unique genomic sequences, one cannot dismiss the possibility that DMBA and MMTV act via a common molecular pathway.
Furthermore, the possibility that DMBA leads to a transient expression
of MMTV has not been addressed in any experiment. Expression of an
endogenous MMTV genomic information may be more important in the initial preneoplastic transformation than in the subsequent neoplastic
transformation. In summary, there are still many unanswered questions
regarding chemical-viral interactions in mammary tumorigenesis. Although the data favor one answer, the emerging cell culture methodology
and viral reagents should allow this question to be addressed in a
more precise and sophisticated fashion than heretofore possible.

REFERENCES

1. Kirschbaum, A., Williams, W. L., and Bittner, J. J., Cancer Res.,
    6:354-362 (1946).

2. Andervont, H. B., and Dunn, T. B., J. Natl. Cancer Inst., 14:329-
    339 (1953).

3. Bonser, G. M., J. Path. Bact., 68:531-546 (1954).

4. Ranadive, K. J., and Hakim, S. A., In: Int. Symp. Mammary Cancer
    (L. Severi, ed.), Perugia, Italy (1958).

5. Biancifori, C., and Caschera, F., *Brit. J. Cancer, 16:*722-730 (1962).

6. Haran-Ghera, N., *Acta Un. Int. Cancer, 19:*765-768 (1963).

7. Faulkin, L. J., Jr., *J. Natl. Cancer Inst., 36:*289-298 (1966).

8. Liebelt, A. G., and Liebelt, R. A., In: Carcinogenesis, A Broad Critique. XX Annual Symp. on Fundamental Cancer Research, University of Texas M.D. Anderson Hospital and Tumor Institute, Williams and Wilkins Co., Baltimore, MD (1967), p. 315-345.

9. Timmermann, A., Bentvelzen, P., Hageman, P. C., and Calafat, J., *J. Gen. Virol., 4:*619-621 (1969).

10. Bentvelzen, P., In: RNA Viruses and Host Genome in Oncogenesis (Emmelot, P. and Bentvelzen, P., eds.), North-Holland Publishing Co., Amsterdam (1972), pp. 309-337.

11. Medina, D., *J. Natl. Cancer Inst., 53:*213-221 (1974).

12. Slemmer, G., *J. Invest. Dermatol., 63:*27-47 (1974).

13. Medina, D. and Warner, M., *J. Natl. Cancer Inst., 57:*331-337 (1976).

14. Hilgers, J. and Bentvelzen, P., *Adv. Cancer Res., 29:*143-195 (1978).

15. Medina, D., *Cancer Res., 36:*2589-2595 (1976).

16. Smith, G. H., Pauley, R. J., Socher, S. H. and Medina, D., *Cancer Res., 38:*4504-4509 (1978).

17. Smith, G. H., Arthur, L. O. and Medina, D., *Int. J. Cancer* (in press) (1980).

18. Medina, D., *J. Natl. Cancer Inst., 57:*1185-1189 (1976).

19. Banerjee, M. R., Wood, B. G. and Washburn, L. L., *J. Natl. Cancer Inst., 53:*1387-1393 (1974).

20. Telang, N. T., Banerjee, M. R., Iyer, A. P. and Kundu, A. B., *Proc. Natl. Acad. Sci., U.S.A., 76:*5886-5890 (1979).

21. Michalides, R., Van Deemter, L., Nusse, R., Ropcke, G., and Boot, I., *J. Virol., 27:*551-559 (1978).

22. Michalides, R., Van Deemter, L., Nusse, R. and Hageman, P., *J. Virol., 31:*63-72 (1979).

23. Medina, D., Butel, J. S., Socher, S. H. and Miller, F. L., *Cancer res., 40*:368-373 (1979).

24. Dusing-Swartz, S., Medina, D., Butel, J. S., and Socher, S. H., *Proc. Natl. Acad. Sci., U.S.A., 79*:5360-5364 (1979).

25. McGrath, C. M., *J. Natl. Cancer Inst., 47*:455-467 (1971).

26. Parks, W. P., Scolnick, E. M., and Kozikowski, E. H., *Science, 184*:158-160 (1974).

27. Pauley, R. J., Medina, D., and Socher, S. H., *J. Virol., 32*:557-566 (1979).

28. Sternberger, L., In: Immunocytochemistry, J. Wiley and Sons, New York (1979), pp. 104-169.

29. St. George, J. A., Cardiff, R. A., Young, L. J. T., and Faulkin, L. J., Jr., *J. Natl. Cancer Inst., 63*:813-820 (1979).

30. Arthur, L. O., Lovenger, G. G., and Schochetmen, G., *J. Virol., 32*:852-859 (1979).

31. Arthur, L. O., Bauer, R. F., Orme, L. S., and Fine, D. L., *Virol., 87*:266-275 (1978).

32. Cohen, J. C., Majors, J. E., and Varmus, H. E., *J. Virol., 32*:483-496 (1979).

A MOLECULAR APPROACH TO STUDIES OF CHEMICAL CARCINOGEN-VIRUS INTERACTION

Raymond V. Gilden
Howard A. Young

Biological Carcinogenesis Program
Frederick Cancer Research Center
Frederick, Maryland

INTRODUCTION

The evaluation of the potential interaction of endogenous retroviral genes and chemical carcinogens requires a detailed knowledge of the number, heterogeneity, and physical location of the viral genes within a species. For purposes of this discussion, we will expand the definition of viruses to those elements which have typical retroviral nucleic acid structures, but which do not occur as encapsidated structures independent of the helper viruses (termed 30S based on sedimentation velocity). Such elements have been found in rats [1,2] and mice [3,4] and preliminary observations have indicated their presence in cats (M. Gonda, unpublished observations). In addition, much current work has led to the generalization that the acute transforming RNA viruses have acquired discrete cellular sequences directly related to the transformation process. Once acquired, these sequences become viral

in the sense that they exist in a stable genetic relationship with
the acquiring virus; however, whether considered in this context or
as genes which exist independently and most probably are important
for normal differentiation processes, they must be considered in the
overall context of chemical-gene interactions. It is possible that
these normal cell genes are the crucial elements in the carcinogenesis
process, the major role of the retroviruses thus being to act as cloning vehicles under the selective pressure of researchers looking for
the rare variant transforming virus. Such an idea renders archaic
the simplistic approach of the past generation which considered the
measurement of a virus per se, as the test of chemical-viral interactions in experimental systems. In this paper we will consider the
current status of the above categories of gene sequences in the rat,
an animal widely used in standard carcinogenesis bioassays and which
(as suggested by one participant of the workshop) appears to be less
plagued by an overabundance of retroviruses than the mouse. With this
information it seems possible to design experiments to test the hypothesis that carcinogenic chemicals may number viral or viral-related
genes among their key targets.

RESULTS

Nontransforming Retroviruses

During the past decade a number of laboratories have reported the isolation of viruses with typical type C morphology from a number of rat
strains. These viruses were found to share a group-specific antigenic
reactivity associated with a major core protein, p27, in both immuno-
diffusion and radioimmunoassay [5,6]. While cell-free passage of
these viruses in vitro could be achieved, titers of rat virus isolates
tend to be low, limited to rat cells, and infectivity is generally
lost on passage. To date, no morphological transformation has been
associated with these viruses either in vitro or in vivo, thus at present they appear to be benign agents. Molecular hybridization experi-

ments have shown related sequences in the DNA of all rat strains tested [7]; however, to date detailed studies of sequence organization, heterogeneity, and intraspecies variation have not been reported. While there is as yet no direct role for these agents in disease processes, they may interact with cellular genes to generate transforming viruses.

30S Retroviral-like Sequences

Many normal rat cell cultures synthesize a RNA species which sediments at 30S under denaturing conditions and which exists as a typical retrovirus-like dimer under nondenaturing conditions. These sequences were found to be associated with the Kirsten and Harvey sarcoma viruses which were isolated after passage of the corresponding mouse leukemia viruses through rats [8,9]. After a varied passage history, solid tumors were produced in mice by cell-free inocula and these tumors yielded the corresponding transforming viruses. These viruses could then transform mouse cells in culture and by appropriate dilution/ selection techniques nonproducer cells were isolated. These nonproducer cells retained the sarcomagenic genome integrated in cell DNA and produced functional transcripts of this genome. These transcripts contained sequences in common with both the original mouse leukemia virus and rat 30S RNA [10,11]. Thus, the initial assumption was that the 30S species contributed the sarcomagenic information to the transforming virus. Several lines of evidence led to early concern with this simple conclusion, i.e., (i) a number of rat type C viruses were found to be mixed populations containing 30S sequence and they themselves were not transforming [12], (ii) normal cells in culture express these sequences independent of a transformed phenotype [13]; (iii) 30S sequences could be "rescued" from rat cells by infection with type C viruses of heterologous species without acquisition of transforming potential [14]; and (iv) the cloned 30S sequence does not transform cells in vitro. Several recent lines of evidence now point to the conclusion that the 30S sequences are not related to transformation, but rather the responsible sequences are cell-derived and have inserted into the 30S genome prior to or during recombination with the helper

virus. Thus, KiSV and HaSV code for a 21K Mr phosphoprotein not found
in cells producing only 30S sequences [15]. Heteroduplex and restriction enzyme analysis both indicate that an insert of approximately
1.1 Kb [16,17] unique to the transforming viruses is found in the 30S
sequences associated with these viruses. Thus, the current structure
of HaSV appears to be 50-100 bases at the 5' end of mouse origin, 900
bases at the 3' end of mouse origin, and an insert of 4.5 Kb of rat
origin distributed in linear order 5' to 3' as approximately 450 bases
30S, 1.1 Kb cellular insert, and the remaining ~3 Kb 30S. KiSV appears
to have a similar structure although the 1.1 Kb cellular insert is
only slightly related to that of HaSV (unpublished observations). In
vitro transformation studies [18] using cloned fragments of HaSV indicate that the portion containing the 1.1 Kb cellular insert is required
for transformation, whereas the 30S sequence 3' to the insert may aug-
ment but are not required for transformation. Other experiments indicate that temperature sensitive transformation mutants have a thermolabile p21 [19]. Thus, at present there is very strong evidence that
p21 is the product of the rat transforming gene and exists in the 1.1
Kb cellular insert described above. Since both KiSV and HaSV produce
an immunologically cross-reactive product, one can assume that the
transforming genes of these viruses are similar, but not necessarily
identical. In fact, evidence of the heterogeneity in these sequences
has been suggested by recent heteroduplex experiments (unpublished
observations). Thus, there may be a family of related sarc genes in
rat cellular DNA and the extent of this variability is an important
area to be elucidated especially in the context of cocarcinogenesis
theories. 30S sequences are found in multiple copies (~25-50) in cell
DNA and, although detailed studies of their physical arrangement remain
to be done, it appears that the HaSV p21 gene is not associated with
30S sequences in normal cellular DNA (R. Ellis and E. Scolnick, unpublished observations). Since we now know that the transforming genome
is a special class of 30S molecule, it appears probable that this normal virus-like structure can undergo recombination with cellular genes,
e.g., sarc, and thus serve as an intermediate in the generation of a
transforming virus. Whether such recombinants can occur naturally

remains to be determined. Conditions in which expression of 30S is
increased, as in early mammary tumors induced by DMBA [20], may increase the probability of such a recombinational event. At this time,
however, a role for 30S sequences in transformation is restricted to
the two cases of generation of interspecies sarcomagenic viruses.

Rat Sarcoma Virus

Rasheed and coworkers [21] reported that cocultivation of a specific
rat cell producing rat type C virus with a chemically transformed rat
cell line having a history of animal passage yielded a transforming
virus (RaSV). This finding has been reproduced [22] and, while other
transformed cells can be substituted for the second cell type, there
is a requirement for the rat type C virus producing cell (designated
SD-1). Neither cell type by itself produces transforming virus nor
can sequences expected for either KiSV or HaSV (i.e., 3' mouse helper
virus) [10,11] be detected or rescued by superinfection with a heterologous virus. Thus, contamination with a known sarcoma virus is effectively ruled out. At the present time a detailed restriction enzyme
map of RaSV is not available, but certain pertinent information is
already in hand. Rat type C virus, but not rat 30S sequences, appear
to be present in RaSV and, strikingly, the virus codes for a 29K Mr
protein cross-reactive with HaSV and KiSV p21 [22]. By analogy with
other transforming viruses and supported by current data, it appears
that RaSV p29 is a fusion protein containing a portion of the NH_2-
terminal gag gene product (p15) and p21. In addition, the transforming
gene of RaSV appears to be highly related to that of HaSV by Southern
blot analysis (R. Ellis, unpublished observations). It would thus
appear that the generation of sarcoma viruses in the rat, as shown
in three separate cases, involved a common or highly related set of
genes. Since RaSV itself does not contain 30S related sequences, but
the two rat cells used in the cocultivation do express 30S sequences,
the recombination of the cellular sarc with viral sequences can evi-
dently occur via different pathways and may involve both type C and
30S sequences as intermediates. Currently, deliberate cell fusion

Conservation of sarc Genes

In keeping with the findings of other transformation-related genes,
the rat sarc appears highly conserved in an evolutionary sense. As
p21 cross-reactivity has been found in a variety of species [23] including man, one would expect the gene to be important for a yet un-
specified function. A biochemical assay utilizing binding to guanine
nucleotides has been developed [24], possibly pointing to a role in
regulatory processes mediated by cyclic nucleotides. In one model
[25] developed for the avian acute leukemia viruses, it has been suggested that the products of transforming genes, present as normal cell
genes, are expressed preferentially in select lineages at specific
times in differentiation. A corresponding viral protein, perhaps modified as the newly acquired sarc evolves to src, could compete for the
function of normal sarc thus preventing further differentiation. We
further speculate that this modification can occur as a result of
fusion such as that producing p29. This hypothesis suggests that cells
producing high levels of sarc transcript or product should be searched
for during embryogenesis. One striking recent result [26] is the discovery of a hemopoietic precursor mouse cell line which produces ten-
fold more p21 than HaSV or KiSV infected cells. It will be of great
importance to generalize these results to other cell systems and to
determine if expression of these endogenous genes occurs during development in vivo.

DISCUSSION

The above constitutes a brief summary of the current status of retroviral and related genes in rats. Current cloning and analytical techniques promise a detailed description of the individual genomes in
rat cell DNA. With this information one can systematically approach
the question of chemical-viral interaction at the molecular level.
The envisioned experiments involve possible molecular rearrangements,
selective transcriptional activation, or preferential binding of

carcinogens to sarc or other genes. An approach to identifying targets of chemical transformation is crucial for the next generation of progress in carcinogenesis research. The above represents one possible beginning, the results of which are not predictable at this time, but should, however, yield definitive results regarding specific sets of gene sequences.

ACKNOWLEDGMENT

This work was supported by Contract No. NO1-CO-75380 with the National Cancer Institute, National Institutes of Health, Bethesda, Maryland 20205.

REFERENCES

1. Tsuchida, N., Shih, M. S., Gilden, R. V., and Hatanaka, M., *J. Virol.*, *14*:1262-1267 (1974).

2. Scolnick, E. M., Goldberg, R. J., and Williams, D., *J. Virol.*, *13*:1211-1219 (1976).

3. Howk, R. S., Troxler, D. H., Lowy, D., Duesberg, P. H., and Scolnick, E. M., *J. Virol.*, *25*:115-123 (1978).

4. Bexmer, P., Olshevsky, U., Baltimore, D., Dolberg, D., and Fan, H., *J. Virol.*, *29*:1168-1176 (1979).

5. Oroszlan, S., Bova, D., Huebner, R. J., and Gilden, R. V., *J. Virol.*, *10*:746-750 (1972).

6. Charman, H. P., White, M. H., Rahman, R., and Gilden, R. V., *J. Virol.*, *17*:51-59 (1976).

7. Anderson, G. R., and Robbins, K. C., *J. Virol.*, *17*:335-351 (1976).

8. Kirsten, W. H., and Mayer, L. A., *J. Natl. Cancer Inst.*, *39*:311-319 (1967).

9. Harvey, J. J., *Nature (London)*, *204*:1104-1105 (1964).

10. Shih, T. Y., Young, H. A., Coffin, J. M., and Scolnick, E. M., *J. Virol.*, *25*:238-252 (1978).

11. Shih, T. Y., Williams, D. R., Weeks, M. O., Maryak, J. M., Vass, W. C., and Scolnick, E. M., *J. Virol.*, *27*:45-55 (1978).

12. Scolnick, E. M., Maryak, J. M., and Parks, W. P., *J. Virol.*, *14*:1435-1444 (1974).

13. Tsuchida, N., Gilden, R. V., and Hatanaka, M., *Proc. Natl. Acad. Sci.*, *U.S.A.*, *71*:4503-4507 (1974).

14. Scolnick, E. M., Vass, W. C., Howk, R. S., and Duesberg, P. H., *J. Virol.*, *29*:964-972 (1979).

15. Shih, T. Y., Weeks, M. O., Young, H. A., and Scolnick, E. M., *Virology*, *96*:64-79 (1979).

16. Young, H. A., Gonda, M. A., DeFeo, D., Ellis, R. W., Nagashima, K., and Scolnick, E. M., *Virology*, in press (1980).

17. Ellis, R. W., DeFeo, D., Maryak, J. M., Young, H. A., Shih, T. Y., Chang, E. H., Lowy, D. R., and Scolnick, E. M., *J. Virol.*, in press (1980).

18. Chang, E. H., Maryak, J. M., Wei, C.-M., Shih, T. Y., Shober, R., Cheung, H. L., Ellis, R. W., Hager, G. L., Scolnick, E. M., and Lowy, D. R., *J. Virol.*, *35*:76-92 (1980).

19. Shih, T. Y., Weeks, M. O., Young, H. A., and Scolnick, E. M., *J. Virol.*, *31*:546-556 (1979).

20. Young, H. A., Wenk, M. L., Goodman, D. G., and Scolnick, E. M., *J. Natl. Cancer Inst.*, *61*:1329-1337 (1978).

21. Rasheed, S., Gardner, M. B., and Huebner, R. J., *Proc. Natl. Acad. Sci.*, *U.S.A.*, *75*:2972-2976 (1978).

22. Young, H. A., Shih, T. Y., Scolnick, E. M., Rasheed, S., and Gardner, M. B., *Proc. Natl. Acad. Sci.*, *U.S.A.*, *76*:3523-3527 (1979).

23. Langebeheim, H., Shih, T. Y., and Scolnick, E. M., *Virology*, in press (1980).

24. Scolnick, E. M., Papageorge, A. G., and Shih, T. Y., *Proc. Natl. Acad. Sci.*, *U.S.A.*, *76*:5355-5359 (1979).

25. Graf, T. H., and Beug, H., *Biochim. Biophys. Acta*, *516*:269-299 (1978).

26. Scolnick, E. M., Weeks, M. O., Shih, T. Y., Ruscetti, S. K., and Dexter, T. M., *Molecular and Cellular Biology*, in press (1981).

MULTI-STAGE RECOMBINATIONAL ORIGIN OF LEUKEMOGENIC VIRUSES DURING THYMIC LYMPHOMA DEVELOPMENT IN MICE EXPOSED TO PHYSICAL AND CHEMICAL CARCINOGENS

Henry S. Kaplan
Alain Decleve*
Miriam Lieberman
Simone Manteuil-Brutlag

Cancer Biology Research Laboratory
Department of Radiology
Stanford University School of Medicine
Stanford, California

INTRODUCTION

It has long been known that mice of many inbred strains (of which strain C57BL/Ka is the most extensively studied) develop a high incidence of lymphomas and lymphatic leukemias following exposure to whole-body x-irradiation or to chemical carcinogens such as the aromatic hydrocarbons, urethan, nitroquinoline oxide, and the nitrosoureas (for references, cf. [38], [39]). Almost all of these tumors arise in the thymus [34,47] and may be prevented by thymectomy [36,52,67]. The tumor cells have been shown to bear typical T-cell markers such as terminal deoxynucleotidyl transferase (TdT) activity and Thy-1, TL, and Ly-1 antigens; they may also express Ly 2,3 [7,26,59,66].

At first, it was presumed that these lymphomas were due to somatic mutation, since it was well established that ionizing radiation and many of the chemical leukemogens are mutagenic. However, the radiation dose-response function proved to be non-linear and had an apparent

---

Current Affiliation: Risk Management Division, Stanford University
School of Medicine, Stanford, California

191

threshold [41]; fractionated exposures at intervals of several days
were more effective than daily fractionation or single exposures [41];
local irradiation of the thymic region alone yielded no tumors [35];
and shielding of one femur during irradiation [40,42], or the injection
of syngeneic bone marrow cells immediately after irradiation [44],
markedly decreased tumor incidence. Somatic mutation was conclusively
eliminated as a possible mechanism when it was discovered that lymphoma
incidence could be restored, in thymectomized irradiated mice, by the
implantation of a histocompatible neonatal thymus graft [43,45] and
that most such tumors arose from the unirradiated cells of the donor
[46,53,54], thus clearly revealing that the mechanism of induction
must be indirect. These observations have recently been repeated and
confirmed in BL 1.1 (Thy 1.1) mice, using thymic grafts from congenic
C57BL/Ka (thy 1.2) donors (M. Lieberman et al., in preparation).

Isolation of Leukemogenic Retroviruses

A possible solution to the paradox of indirect induction was suggested
by Gross's report [17] that cell-free extracts prepared from thymic
lymphomas arising "spontaneously" in the high-leukemia AKR strain were
leukemogenic when inoculated into newborn mice of the low-leukemia C3H
strain. When cell-free extracts were similarly prepared from thymic
lymphomas arising in irradiated C57BL/Ka mice and inoculated into nonirradiated syngeneic newborns, the latter developed a low but significantly elevated incidence of thymic lymphomas after a long latent period decreased with serial passage of such extracts [37,56,60]. In
time, the leukemogenic agent was shown to have the properties of a
type C retrovirus, and named the radiation leukemia virus (RadLV).
These findings were later confirmed by other investigators [1,19,33,
51,79].

Moreover, reports began to emerge indicating that the thymic lymphomas induced in various murine strains by the chemical carcinogens
also contained subcellular leukemogenic agents with the attributes
of type C retroviruses [3,4,20,31,32,50,69,73,78], though negative

results have been reported in other studies [23,48,68,70]. Perhaps
the most convincing evidence was provided by Ball and McCarter [3],
who found that cell-free filtrates as well as suspensions or supernatants of lethally irradiated tumor cells from 9 of 11 consecutive
thymic lymphomas induced in CFW/D mice by a single neonatal injection
of 7,12-dimethylbenz(a)anthracene (DMBA) yielded identical tumors after
direct intrathymic inoculation into neonatal or thymic graft-bearing
syngeneic mice. Serial animal passage of a cell-free filtrate from
a transplanted DMBA-induced lymphoma resulted in an increase of tumor
incidence to 60% by the third passage.

When RadLV was injected directly into one lobe of the thymus of
neonatal or infant mice, histological evidence of lymphoma development
was consistently observed first in the injected lobe, and the spread
of tumor cells to the contralateral lobe was a secondary event [21].
This simple experiment proved that RadLV acts directly to transform
thymic cells, and excludes the possibility of indirect mechanisms involving viral alteration of hormonal or other systemic regulatory functions. Moreover, three lines of evidence strongly suggest that information carried by the virus is implicated in the etiology of the thymic
lymphomas which develop in mice exposed to fractionated whole-body
x-irradiation; (1) the thymic implant experiments cited previously
[43,45,46,53,54] demonstrated that these tumors are not the direct
consequence of irradiation; (2) primary radiation-induced thymic lymphomas of C57BL/Ka and BALB/c mice can absorb cytotoxic antibodies
prepared in W/Fu rats against RadLV-induced rat lymphomas, indicating
that the radiogenic and virogenic lymphomas must share cell membrane
antigenic determinants [15]; (3) inoculation of C57BL/Ka mice with
syngeneic embryo fibroblasts infected by and continuously producing
BL/Ka(B), a B-ecotropic, nonleukemogenic virus, was found to confer
immunity against the transplantation of syngeneic lymphomas, and to
partially protect such mice against the induction of thymic lymphomas
by either RadLV or X rays [61]. Immunoprevention of radiogenic lymphoma development in C57BL mice has also been achieved by active immunization with Rauscher murine leukemia virus (MuLV) and by passive
immunization with goat antibody to Gross MuLV [71].

Collectively, these observations suggested that leukemogenic retroviruses may be involved in the genesis of most or all murine thymic lymphomas, irrespective of the external inducing agent. Our initial hypothesis, now known to be incorrect, was that the genomes of such viruses pre-exist in biologically inert, "latent" form, and are triggered to an "activated" state by radiation or chemicals, by some mechanism presumably akin to that of the induction of temperate bacteriophage in lysogenic bacteria [64].

Properties of RadLV and Other C57BL/Ka Retroviral Isolates

RadLV has been extensively characterized with respect to its biological and serologic properties [8,9]. It is highly leukemogenic (L+), inducing lymphomas after direct intrathymic inoculation at titers as high as 10^9/ml, and highly thymotropic (T+), as measured by the rapid and selective expression of viral antigens in lymphoid cells of the thymic cortex after intravenous or intrathymic inoculation [11,12]. However, it shows little or no capacity to replicate in syngeneic mouse embryo fibroblasts (fibrotropism; F-), except at high multiplicities of infection ([11], Decleve et al., manuscript in preparation). Since it could not be grown in vitro on fibroblasts, this T+L+F-virus has been propagated for more than 20 years by serial blind thymic passage in pre-weaning C57BL/Ka mice. More recently, several permanent cell lines established in culture from RadLV-induced C57BL/Ka thymic lymphomas were all found to produce virus promptly and continuously during serial in vitro passage [59]. The virus produced by the BL/VL$_3$ cell line, designated RadLV/VL$_3$, was found to have thymotropic and leukemogenic activity as well as other properties essentially indistinguishable from those of the parental RadLV virus [10]. Since RadLV/VL$_3$ virus can be conveniently harvested from BL/VL$_3$ cultures in high titer, it has been used in recent studies of the viral genome [65] and of the virion structural proteins [16].

Meanwhile, three other types of retroviruses have been isolated from normal or neoplastic tissues of C57BL/Ka mice [8,56,62]. All three are devoid of thymotropic of leukemogenic activity, but replicate well on fibroblasts of appropriate genotype, and are thus classi-

fied as T-L-F+. One of these, BL/Ka(B), replicates preferentially on
Fv-1^{bb} cells; BL/Ka(N) is also ecotropic, but replicates preferentially
on Fv-1^{nn} cells; and BL/Ka(X), though readily expressed by normal and
neoplastic murine thymocytes, replicates only on non-murine fibroblasts
and is thus xenotropic [55].

When the virion proteins of RadLV were radioiodinated and analyzed
by SDS-polyacrylamide gel electrophoresis (SDS-PAGE), they revealed
a pattern generally similar to that of the Moloney murine leukemia
virus: an envelope glycoprotein of about 70,000 daltons (gp70), a major
internal core protein of 30,000 daltons (p30), and three small polypeptides of 10,000 to 15,000 daltons (p15, p12, and p10;81). Antibodies
against the virus readily detect the p30 in the cytoplasm and the gp70
at the surface membrane of infected cells, using indirect immunofluorescence [11,12]. Neutralization, immunofluorescence and competition
radioimmunoassay (RIA) methods demonstrated that the gp70 of RadLV is
serologically distinguishable from those of BL/Ka(B),-(N), and -(X),
and that RadLV cannot be neutralized by antibodies to the gp70's of
other ecotropic viruses and is only partially neutralizable by high
titer antibody to xenotropic virus gp70 [8,9].

Tryptic digest peptide maps of the RadLV gp70 (J.H. Elder et al.,
unpublished) provided evidence that it is apparently a recombinant
molecule derived from the gp70's of BL/Ka(N) and BL/Ka(X), as is that
of BL/Ka(B). Peptide mapping and RIA studies [16] have now shown that
the p30 of RadLV is also derived by recombination of the corresponding
polypeptides of BL/Ka(N) and BL/Ka(X). The simplest interpretation
is that RadLV was derived from a recombinational event in which an insert of the xenotropic virus extending from the region of the gag gene
which codes for the p30 through the entire pol gene and a part of the
env gene region displaces the corresponding regions of the BL/Ka(N)
genome. Competition radioimmunoassay studies [5] indicate that the
B-tropic non-leukemogenic BL/Ka(B) viral genome is also derived by
recombination of two endogenous C57BL/Ka viruses, BL/Ka(N) and BL/Ka(X).
The possibility that the recombinational event(s) leading to the formation of the RadLV and BL/Ka(B) genomes occurred at some time in the
distant past and that they are now carried by strain C57BL/Ka mice

as additional endogenous proviruses cannot be excluded on present evidence, but seems unlikely in view of molecular hybridization studies
[28] indicating the presence of only one endogenous ecotropic viral
locus in backcrosses involving the related C57BL/6 strain.

Paradoxical Absence of Viral Antigens after Irradiation

The hypothesis that RadLV emerges after a single-step "activation" of
a biologically inert provirus would have predicted that viral antigens
should appear in the relevant target tissues (thymus, bone marrow,
and/or spleen) promptly after irradiation. When specific serologic
reagents became available, this prediction was tested. In striking
contrast to the rapid appearance of viral antigens in the cortical
thymocytes after intrathymic or intravenous inoculation of RadLV [11,
12], immunofluorescence tests sensitive enough to have detected one
antigen-positive cell in 20,000-40,000 cells failed to reveal any viral
antigen-positive cells in the thymuses of C57BL/Ka mice at intervals
ranging from one week to two months after fractionated whole-body x-
irradiation [62]. Even at 4 months after x-irradiation, when lymphomas
were evident in most thymuses, only 19 percent of such thymuses in
an initial study [62], and even fewer (about 5 percent) in more extensive studies, were found to contain antigen-psoitive cells, and even
in these few, only 0.01-0.05% of cells were positive [56]. Antibody
studies [29,30] have also failed to reveal consistent evidence of ecotropic retrovirus expression in the tissues of irradiated C57BL mice.
However, infectivity assays have indicated the transient production
of a virus with the properties of BL/Ka(B) within the first several
days after irradiation, followed thereafter by the disappearance of
infectious virus [18].

Yet, cell-free extracts of autochthonous C57BL/Ka thymic lymphomas
developing after fractionated whole-body x-irradiation [37,60], as
well as serial in vivo transplants [56] or in vitro subpassages [59]
of such lymphomas, have repeatedly been found to contain leukemogenic
virus when assayed by direct intrathymic inoculation in infant C57BL/Ka
mice, whereas similarly prepared extracts of normal C57BL/Ka thymus,

spleen, or bone marrow are devoid of leukemogenic activity. When cell-free extracts were prepared and assayed at various intervals during the preneoplastic period, leukemogenic virus was not detectable in the thymus of C57BL/Ka mice until two months after irradiation and then only at low levels [56,60]. However, the transient presence of leukemogenic virus in the bone marrow of strain C57BL/6 mice about one week after x-irradiation has been reported [22].

   The time of first expression of leukemogenic virus varies even in fully developed thymic lymphomas. In one study, leukemogenic activity was present in extracts prepared from 7 of 10 consecutive autochthonous lymphomas of irradiated C57BL/Ka mice [37]. In a later study, five such lymphomas which were devoid of leukemogenic virus in the original animal all became positive for leukemogenic viral activity during the course of serial transplantation in syngeneic hosts; some were positive at the first in vivo passage, others not until the second or third passage [56,60]. Permanent cell lines of radiogenic C57BL/Ka thymic lymphomas have also been established in vitro; although 5 of 8 such cell lines ultimately expressed cytoplasmic viral antigens, only one did so within one month in culture, a second after two months, sublines of two others after three months, and one cell line not until two years. Three cell lines (BL/RL_{11}, $_{-14}$, and $_{-17}$) and sublines of two others (BL/RL_{10}-NP and BL/RL_{12}-NP) have remained antigen negative for more than two years in culture [59]. Cell lines and sublines that became virus-positive continued indefinitely thereafter to produce virus. When the viral isolates from three of these cell lines were assayed in vivo, they were found to share with RadLV the properties of thymotropism and leukemogenicity [59].

   The fact that cytoplasmic viral antigen expression and virus production are consistently absent in the thymuses, and even in fully developed thymic lymphomas, of irradiated C57BL/Ka mice, whereas RadLV and $RadLV/VL_3$ are highly thymotropic, made it necessary to abandon the original hypothesis that RadLV exists as an endogenous proviral genome in the cellular DNA of this strain and is directly "activated" by exposure to radiation and/or chemical carcinogens. Instead, the hypothesis was proposed [9] that radiation induces the expression of

a subviral entity which is endowed with the capacity for neoplastic
transformation of the murine thymocyte(s) in which it develops but is
replication defective. It was suggested that at a later stage, usually
after a frank thymic lymphoma has developed, this subviral entity is
converted to the replication-competent infectious, thymotropic and
leukemogenic retrovirus, RadLV.

A direct test of this hypothesis became possible when it was discovered that the BL/RL_{12}-NP subline, which has remained completely
devoid of viral antigen expression and virus production during more
than three years in culture [59], was not only highly permissive for
infection by RadLV and $RadLV/VL_3$, thus providing the basis for a con-
venient in vitro assay system [58], but also moderately permissive
for the BL/Ka(B) virus, though not for BL/Ka(N) or BL/Ka(X). It was
of interest that the BL/Ka(B) virus, though unable to replicate in
the normal thymocytes of adult C57BL/Ka mice, was able to do so in
neoplastic thymocytes. Even more interesting was the observation, in
6 of 10 consecutive experiments, that the progeny virus emerging from
BL/Ka(B) infected BL/RL_{12}-NP cells had acquired thymotropism and leukemogenicity, properties entirely lacking in the parental virus [57].
In some instances, these properties were stable during serial in vivo
passage, whereas in others they were lost. That the emergent progeny
virus was not identical with RadLV was evident from the fact that,
like BL/Ka(B), it could readily be neutralized with antibody to ecotropic virus gp71 and had a moderate degree of fibrotropism. It was
therefore concluded that oncogenic (T+L+) sequences endogenous to the
nonproducer lymphoma cells had been packaged as virus-like particles
as a consequence of infection by a T-L- virus, presumably by recombinational or helper-rescue mechanisms, leading to the production of
true recombinants, phenotypically mixed particles, heterozygotes, and/
or a mixed population of helper BL/Ka(B) and defective T+L+ particles.

It is clear that the rescue of T+L+ particles could not have
occurred if T+L+ sequences had not pre-existed in the $BLRL_{12}$-NP cells.
Thus, the rescue of these sequences provided strong support for the
subviral entity hypothesis. This defective genome presumably induces
and maintains the transformed phenotype in the neoplastic thymocytes

of irradiated C57BL/Ka mice, but fails to produce detectable amounts of the major virion structural proteins, p30 and gp70, or of free virus. These neoplastic thymocytes, like BL/RL$_{12}$-NP cells, may be permissive for in vivo superinfection by BL/Ka(B) virus, expressed randomly in the thymus and/or bone marrow of tumor-bearing mice, leading to the emergence of a replication-competent T+L+ population of virus particles. The other distinctive properties of RadLV, such as its unique gp70 and augmented leukemogenicity, may have been acquired as a consequence of selection during more than 20 years of serial blind thymic passage in vivo.

Further strong support for these concepts has come from comparative studies of the RadLV/VL$_3$ and the BL/Ka(B) viral genomes [65]. When analyzed on agarose gels under denaturing conditions, RadLV/VL$_3$ preparations were found to contain equimolar amounts of two high molecular weight RNAs, 8.0 $\pm$ 0.3 and 5.6 $\pm$ 0.2 kilobases (Kb) in length, both of which could be biosynthetically labeled with ^{3}H-uridine. In contrast, the BL/Ka(B) virus contained a single high molecular weight RNA species of 8.0 $\pm$ 0.3 Kb, but no detectable 5.6 Kb RNA. The fact that these high molecular weight RNAs bound to oligo(dT)-cellulose indicated that they contain poly(A). When RadLV/VL$_3$ RNA was analyzed on velocity gradients, two major species sedimenting at 70 S and 54 S were resolved. After denaturation, the sedimentation velocities of these molecules decreased to 38 S and 31 S, in keeping with expectation for monomeric RNAs 8 Kb and 5.6 Kb in lenght. The 70 S and 54 S species present in the virions are thus dimers, similar to those described for other retroviruses [6,13,74]. The "melting" profiles of the 70 S and 54 S dimers were indistinguishable, indicating that their dimer linkage structures [6] have identical stabilities.

The 70 S and 54 S RNAs were both able to serve as primer templates for the reverse transcriptase of avian myeloblastosis virus. For both templates, the major reaction product was a cDNA 147 $\pm$ 1 bases long (strong-stop DNA, ssDNA; ref. 24). The patterns of DNA fragments smaller than 147 bases were also indistinguishable. Moreover, ssDNA made from either template hybridized to the same extent to the 8.0 Kb monomers. Thus, the 5' termini of the 8.0 and 5.6 Kb monomers must have closely similar or identical sequences.

In cells producing retroviruses with the genomic structure 5'-
gag-pol-env-3', two species of viral RNA, with properties similar to
those of messenger RNA's, have been detected: a 35 S species corresponding in length to the complete viral genome and believed to serve
as the gag-pol messenger [72], and a 21 S species which contains a
short sequence from the 5' terminus spliced onto the 3' third of the
genome and is thought to encode the env gene translation product [75].
When poly(A)-containing cytoplasmic RNA from BL/VL$_3$ cells was examined
for the presence of viral-specific sequences, four RNA species with
lengths of 8.0, 5.6, 3.4, and 1.6 Kb were detected. By analogy with
other retroviruses, it seemed likely that the 8.0 and 5.6 Kb RNAs are
similar to the two high molecular weight RNA species found in RadLV/VL$_3$
virions. If so, the 8.0 Kb species may be presumed to code for the
gag and pol precursor proteins; the function of the 5.6 Kb species
remains to be determined. A randomly primed cDNA prepared from the
BL/Ka(B) 8.0 Kb RNA did not hybridize detectably with the 1.6 Kb RNA
species, the function of which also remains unknown.

The major protein products were identified when either the 8.0
Kb or the 5.6 Kb viral RNAs were used as templates for in vitro translation. The 8 Kb RNA produced 63,000 and 70,000 dalton proteins similar in size to those produced by in vitro translation of Moloney MuLV
RNA [14,49]. Proteins of the same sizes were also synthesized in vitro
from the 8.0 Kb RNA of BL/Ka(B) virus. These are believed to be, respectively, the gag precursor polyprotein and a glycosylated product
expressed at the surface of infected cells. The major products of
translation of the 5.6 Kb RNA were 36,000 and 30,000 dalton proteins.
These products were immunoprecipitable with a combination of antibodies
directed against the Gross-AKR MuLV p12 and p14 proteins (α-p12 +
α-p14). In addition, a 100,000 dalton minor translation product of
the 5.6 Kb RNA was a major constituent of the proteins immunoprecipi-
tated by α-p12 + α-p14. None of the 5.6 Kb RNA translation products
were immunoprecipitable by antibody to Gross-AKR MuLV p30. It was
concluded that the 5.6 Kb RNA of RadLV/VL$_3$ contains p15 and p12 gene

sequences but few or no p30 sequences, and that it codes for a 100,000 dalton polyprotein containing gag antigenic determinants.

The 5.6 Kb genome of RadLV/VL$_3$ thus appears to be structurally similar at its 5' end to that of the Abelson murine leukemia virus (A-MuLV; ref. 76). If so, it may be suggested that the 8.0 Kb RNA species of RadLV/VL$_3$ is that of a replication-competent helper virus, and that the 5.6 Kb species represents a defective recombinant genome which codes for a transforming gene product but not for p30 or gp70. Thus, its intracellular expression could initiate and maintain the transformed phenotype, but would not yield cytoplasmic antigens detectable by antibodies directed against either of these major virior structural proteins.

The 8,0 Kb and 5.6 Kb proviral DNAs of RadLV/VL$_3$ have now been tentatively identified in freshly infected BL/RL$_{12}$-NP cells and are being cloned in bacterial hosts, using recombinant DNA techniques. Once these cloned DNA probes become available, it should readily be possible to ascertain whether sequences homologous to the 5.6 Kb genome are present in all C57BL/Ka thymic lymphomas. If so, it will be of interest to determine how soon after fractionated whole-body irradiation such sequences can be detected in target cells for neoplastic transformation. It will also become possible to test the hypothesis that a 3.0 Kb insert in the 5.6 Kb genome which is non-homologous to the 8.0 Kb viral RNA is derived from normal cellular sequences.

A replication-defective, transformation-competent subviral entity could have been generated by mechanisms similar to those postulated in the "promoter insertion" hypothesis, for which evidence has recently been put forward by Shimotohno et al [77], Hayward [25], and Vande Woude [80]. If so, it may be speculated that specific normal cellular sequences recombined or underwent splicing, soon after irradiation, with the 5' long terminal repeat (LTR) and part of the gag gene of a transiently expressed endogenous helper virus such as BL/Ka(B). This replication-defective entity could have initiated and maintained the neoplastic transformation of thymic target cells, in the complete absence of viral expression or replication, until rescued by a second recombinational event following superinfection of the tumor cells with

a BL/Ka(B)-like virus. Infectious, leukemogenic virus would then become extractable from the tumor-bearing tissues of its murine host.

It may also be possible to accommodate within this hypothesis
the fact that mice of certain strains such as C57L(2) and NIH/Swiss
(Lieberman et al., Ihle et al., unpublished) are susceptible to radiation-induced thymic lymphoma development despite the fact that they
harbor xenotropic but no detectable ecotropic endogenous viral genomes
[63]. In such strains, it is possible that the 5' or 3' LTR of the
endogenous xenotropic virus, after irradiation, can serve as the vector
for inverting the corresponding cellular sequences into target cell
DNA. The resultant lymphomas would not be expected to yield leukemogenic viruses even after extensive serial transplantation or in vitro
culture both because they lack ecotropic viruses and because rescue
by an ecotropic virus would be difficult or impossible if, as seems
likely, there is a lack of homology between the LTR's of ecotropic
and xenotropic viruses. In this situation, it is possible that lymphoma cell genomes would contain oncogenic cellular sequences similar
to those in producer lymphomas, linked to sequences homologous to the
LTR's of xenotropic virus, a prediction which will soon also be subject
to test. We may therefore be approaching the time when definitive
evidence can be provided to define the respective roles of cellular
sequences and of viral 5' or 3' insertion sequences in the development
of thymic lymphomas, and to trace the recombinational events leading
to the genesis of the leukemogenic viruses they may contain, in susceptible murine strains exposed to ionizing radiation or to chemical
carcinogens.

ACKNOWLEDGMENT

The work from this laboratory cited here was supported in part by
grants CA-03352 and CA-25619 from the National Cancer Institute,
National Institutes of Health.

REFERENCES

1. Ageenko, A. I., Leukemogenic agent isolated from irradiated C57BL
    mice, *Probl. Hematol.*, *7*:8-13, (1962).

2. Arnstein, P., Riggs, J. L., Oshiro, L. S., Huebner, R. J., and
    Lennette, E. M., Production of lymphomia and associated xenotroph-
    ic type-C virus in C57L mice by whole-body irradiation, *J. Natl.
    Cancer Inst.*, *57*:1085-1090, (1976).

3. Ball, J. K. and McCarter, J. A., Repeated demonstration of a mouse
    leukemia virus after treatment with chemical carcinogens, *J. Natl.
    Cancer Inst.*, *46*:751-762, (1971).

4. Basombrio, M. A., Lymphomas in BALB/c mice inoculated with super-
    natants from chemically induced sarcomas, *J. Natl. Cancer Inst.*,
    51:1157-1162, (1973).

5. Benade, L. E., Ihle, J. N., and Decleve, A., Serological charac-
    terization of B-tropic viruses of C57BL mice: possible origin
    by recombination of endogenous N-tropic and xenotropic viruses,
    Proc. Natl. Acad. Sci., *U.S.A.-Microbiology, 75*:4553-4557, (1978).

6. Bender, W., Chien, Y. H., Chattopadhyay, S., Vogt, P. K., Gardner,
    M. B., and Davidson, N., High-molecular-weight RNAs of AKR NZB,
    and wild mouse viruses and avian reticuloendotheliosis virus all
    have similar dimer structures, *J. Virol.*, *25*:888-896, (1978).

7. Chazan, R., and Haran-Ghera, N., The role of thymus subpopulations
    in "T" leukemia development, *Cell Immunol.*, *23*:3257-375,(1976).

8. Decleve, A., Lieberman, M., Ihle, J. N., and Kaplan, H. S., Bio-
    logical and serological characterization of radiation leukemia
    virus (RadLV), *Proc. Natl. Acad. Sci.*, *U.S.A.*, *73*:4675-4679,
    (1976).

9. Decleve, A., Lieberman, M., Ihle, J. N., and Kaplan, H. S., Bio-
    logical and serological characterization of the C-type RNA viruses
    isolated from the C57BL/Ka strain of mice. In: J. F. Duplan
    (ed.), Radiation-Induced Leukemogenesis and Related Viruses,
    pp. 247-264. Amsterdam: North-Holland Pub., 1977.

10. Decleve, A., Lieberman, M., Ihle, J. N., Rosenthal, P. N., Lung,
    M. L., and Kaplan, H. S., Physicochemical, biological and sero-
    logical properties of a leukemogenic virus isolated from cultured
    RadLV-induced lymphomas of C57BL/Ka mice, *Virology, 90*:23-35,
    (1978).

11. Decleve, A., Sato, C., Lieberman, M., and Kaplan, H. S., Selective
    thymic localization of murine leukemia virus-related antigens
    in C57BL/Ka mice after inoculation with radiation leukemia virus,
    Proc. Natl. Acad. Sci., *U.S.A.*, *71*:3124-3128, 1974.

12. Decleve, A., Travis, M., Weissman, I. L., Lieberman, M., and
     Kaplan, H. S., Focal infection and transformation in situ of thy-
     mic cell subclasses by a thymotropic murine leukemia virus, *Cancer
     Res.*, *35*:3585-3595, (1975).

13. Dube, S., Kung, H.-J., Bender, W., Davidson, N., and Ostertag, W.,
     Size, subunit composition, and secondary structure of the Friend
     virus genome, *J. Virol.*, *20*:264-272, (1976).

14. Edwards, S. A. and Fan, H., Gag-related polyproteins of Moloney
     murine leukemia virus: evidence for independent synthesis of gly-
     cosylated and unglycosylated forms, *J. Virol.*, *30*:551-563, (1979).

15. Ferrer, J. F. and Kaplan, H. S., Antigenic characteristics of lym-
     phomas induced by radiation leukemia virus (RadLV) in mice and
     rats, *Cancer Res.*, *28*:2522-2528, (1968).

16. Goodenow, R., Olcott, E., Decleve, A., Lieberman, M., and Kaplan,
     H. S., Evidence for type-specific antigenic sites on the p30 of
     radiation leukemia virus, Cold Spring Harbor RNA Tumor Virus
     Symposium, 1980 (abstr.).

17. Gross, L., "Spontaneous" leukemia developing in C3H mice following
     inoculation, in infancy, with AK-leukemic extracts, or AK-embryo,
     Proc. Soc. Exp. Biol. Med., *76*:27-32, (1951).

18. Haas, M., Transient virus expression during murine leukemia induc-
     tion by x-irradiation, *J. Natl. Cancer Inst.*, *58*:251-257, (1977).

19. Haran-Ghera, N., Leukemogenic activity of centrifuges from irradi-
     ated mouse thymus and bone marrow, *Int. J. Cancer, 1*:81-87,
     (1966).

20. Haran-Ghera, N., A leukemogenic filtrable agent from chemically-
     induced lymphoid leukemia in C57BL mice, *Proc. Soc. Exp. Biol.
     Med., 124*:697-699, (1967).

21. Haran-Ghera, N., Lieberman, M., and Kaplan, H. S., Direct action
     of a leukemogenic virus on the thymus, *Cancer Res.*, *26*:438-441,
     (1966).

22. Haran-Ghera, N. and Peled, A., The mechanism of radiation action
     in leukemogenesis. Isolation of a leukemogenic filtrable agent
     from tissues of irradiated and normal C57BL mice, *Br. J. Cancer,
     21*:730-738, (1967).

23. Harvey, J. J., East, J., and Katz, F. E., Azathioprine-induced
     lymphocytic neoplasms of NZB mice lack ecotropic murine leukemia
     virus, *Int. J. Cancer, 23*:217-223, (1979).

24. Haseltine, W. A., Kleid, D. G., Panet, A., Rothenberg, E., and
     Baltimore, D., Ordered transcription of RNA tumor virus genomes,
     J. Mol. Biol., 106:109-131, (1976).

25. Hayward, W. S., Avian lymphoid leukosis is correlated with the appearance of discrete new RNAs containing viral and cellular genetic information; leukemogenesis by promoter insertion? In: R. Neth and K. Mannweiler (eds.), Modern Trends in Leukemia IV, Berlin: Springer-Verlag, in press.

26. Hiai, H., Shisa, H., Matsudaira, Y., and Nishizuka, Y., Theta antigen in N-mitrosobutylurea leukemogenesis of the mouse, *Gann*, *64*:197-201, (1973).

27. Igel, H. J., Huebner, R. J., Turner, H. C., Kotin, P., and Falk, H. L., Mouse leukemia virus activation by chemical carcinogens, *Science*, *166*:1624-1626, (1969).

28. Ihle, J. N. and Joseph, D. R., Genetic analysis of the endogenous C3H murine leukemia virus genome: evidence for one locus unlinked to the endogenous murine leukemia virus genome of C57BL/6 mice, *Virology*, *87*:298-306, (1978).

29. Ihle, J. N., Joseph, D. R., and Pazmino, N. H., Radiation leukemia in C57BL/6 mice. II. Lack of ecotropic virus expression in the majority of lymphomas, *J. Exp. Med.*, *144*:1406-1423, (1976).

30. Ihle, J. N., McEwan, R., and Bengali, K., Radiation leukemia in C57BL/6 mice. I. Lack of serological evidence for the role of endogenous viruses in pathogenesis, *J. Exp. Med.*, *144*:1391-1405, (1976).

31. Imamura, N., Evidence of viral implication in experimental leukemia induced by N-nitrosobutylurea in mice, *Gann*, *64*:47-57, (1973).

32. Irino, S., Ota, Z., Sezaki, T., Suzaki, M., and Hiraki, K., Cell-free transmission of 20-methylcholanthrene-induced RF mouse leukemia and electron microscopic demonstration of virus particles in its leukemic tissue, *Gann*, *54*:225-237, (1963).

33. Irino, S., Sota, S., and Hiraki, K., The role of virus in radiation leukemogenesis, *Gann*, *57*:507-511, (1966).

34. Kaplan, H. S., Comparative susceptibility of lymphoid tissues of strain C57 black mice to induction of lymphoid tumors by irradiation, *J. Natl. Cancer Inst.*, *8*:191-197, (1948).

35. Kaplan, H. S., Preliminary studies of the effectiveness of local irradiation in the induction of lymphoid tumors in mice, *J. Natl. Cancer Inst.*, *10*:267-270, (1949).

36. Kaplan, H. S., Influence of thymectomy, splenectomy and gonadectomy on incidence of radiation-induced lymphoid tumors in strain C57 black mice, *J. Natl. Cancer Inst.*, *11*:83-90, (1950).

37. Kaplan, H. S., On the natural history of the murine leukemias: presidential address, *Cancer Res.*, *27*:1325-1340, (1967).

38. Kaplan, H. S., Leukemia and lymphoma in experimental and domestic animals, *Ser. Haemat.*, *7*:94-163, (1974).

39. Kaplan, H. S., Etiology of lymphomas and leukemias: Role of C-type RNA viruses, *Leuk. Res.*, *2*:253-271, (1978).

40. Kaplan, H. S. and Brown, M. B., Further observations on inhibition of lymphoid tumor development by shielding and partial body irradiation of mice, *J. Natl. Cancer Inst.*, *12*:427-436, (1951).

41. Kaplan, H. S. and Brown, M. B., A quantitative dose-response study of lymphoid-tumor development in irradiated C57 black mice, *J. Natl. Cancer Inst.*, *13*:185-208, (1952).

42. Kaplan, H. S. and Brown, M. B., Protection against radiation-induced lymphoma development by shielding and partial body irradiation of mice, *Cancer Res.*, *12*:441-444, (1952).

43. Kaplan, H. S. and Brown, M. B., Development of lymphoid tumors in nonirradiated thymic grafts in thymectomized irradiated mice., *Science*, *119*:439-440, (1954).

44. Kaplan, H. S., Brown, M. B., and Paull, J., Influence of bone marrow injections on involution and neoplasia of mouse thymus after systemic irradiation, *J. Natl. Cancer Inst.*, *14*:303-316, (1953).

45. Kaplan, H. S., Carnes, W. H., Brown, M. B., and Hirsch, B. B., Indirect induction of lymphomas in irradiated mice. I. Tumor incidence and morphology in mice bearing nonirradiated thymic grafts, *Cancer Res.*, *16*:422-425, (1956).

46. Kaplan, H. S., Hirsch, B. B., and Brown, M. B., Indirect induction of lymphomas in irradiated mice. IV. Genetic evidence of the origin of the tumor cells from the thymic grafts, *Cancer Res.*, *16*:434-436, (1956).

47. Kaplan, H. S. and Lieberman, M., The role of lymphoid and haematopoietic target cells in viral lymphomagenesis of C57BL/Ka mice. II. Neoplastic transformation of bone marrow-derived cells in the thymic microenvironment, *Blood Cells*, *2*:301-317, (1976).

48. Kawamura, Y., Type-C RNA viruses and leukemogenesis: relation of type-C virus infectivity and leukemogenesis induced by nitrosourea compounds in mice, *Gann*, *67*:389-398, (1976).

49. Kerr, I. M., Olshevsky, U., Lodish, H. F., and Baltimore, D., Translation of murine leukemia virus RNA in cell-free systems from animals cells, *J. Virol.*, *18*:627-635, (1976).

50. Kinosita, R. and Tanaka, T., Lymphoma in ICR mice treated with 4-nitroquinoline oxide (4NQO). In: Viruses, Nucleic Acids, and Cancer, Univ. of Texas M. D. Anderson Hospital Tumor Institute, Baltimore: Williams and Wilkins Co., pp. 571-574, 1963.

51. Latarjet, R. and Duplan, J.-F., Experiment and discussion on leukemogenesis by cell-free extracts of radiation-induced luekaemia in mice, *Int. J. Radiat. Biol.*, 5:339-344, (1962).

52. Law, L. W., and Miller, J. H., Observations on the effect of thymectomy in spontaneous leukemias in mice of the high-leukemia strains RIL and C58, *J. Natl. Cancer Inst.*, 11:253-262, (1950).

53. Law, L. W. and Potter, M., The behavior in transplant of lymphocytic neoplasms arising from parental thymic grafts in irradiated, thymectomized hybrid mice, *Proc. Natl. Acad. Sci.*, *U.S.A.*, 42:160-167, (1956).

54. Law, L. W. and Potter, M., Further evidence of indirect induction by x-radiation of lymphocytic neoplasms in mice, *J. Natl. Cancer Inst.*, 20:489-493, (1958).

55. Levy, J. A., Xenotropic viruses: murine leukemia viruses associated with NIH Swiss, NZB, and other mouse strains, *Science*, 182:1151-1153, (1973).

56. Lieberman, M., Decleve, A., Gelmann, E. P., and Kaplan, H. S., Biological and serological characterization of the C-type RNA viruses isolated from the C57BL/Ka strain of mice. II. Induction and propagation of the isolates. In: Radiation-Induced Leukemogenesis and Related Viruses, J. F. Duplan (ed.), pp. 231-246, Amsterdam: North-Holland Pub., 1977.

57. Lieberman, M., Decleve, A., Ihle, J. N., and Kaplan, H. S., Rescue of a thymotropic, leukemogenic C-type virus from cultured, nonproducer lymphoma cells of strain C57BL/Ka mice, *Virology, 97*:12-21, (1979).

58. Lieberman, M., Decleve, A., and Kaplan, H. S., Rapid in vitro assay for thymotropic, leukemogenic murine C-type RNA viruses, *Virology, 90*:274-278, (1978).

59. Lieberman, M., Decleve, A., Ricciardi-Castagnoli, P., Boniver, J., Finn, O. J., and Kaplan, H. S., Establishment, characterization, and virus expression of cell lines derived from radiation- and virus-induced lymphomas of C57BL/Ka mice, *Int. J. Cancer, 24*:168-177, (1979).

60. Lieberman, M. and Kaplan, H. S., Leukemogenic activity of filtrates from radiation-induced lymphoid tumors of mice, *Science, 130*:387-388, (1959).

61. Lieberman, M. and Kaplan, H. S., Vaccination against x-ray or radiation leukemia virus-induced thymic lymphoma development by inoculation of mice with syngeneic fibroblastic cells infected with an endogenous B-tropic nonleukemogenic virus. In: Radiation-Induced Leukemogenesis and Related Viruses, J. D. Duplan (ed.), pp. 127-132, Amsterdam: North-Holland Pub., 1977.

62. Lieberman, M., Kaplan, H. S., and Decleve, A., Anomalous viral expression in radiogenic lymphomas of C57BL/Ka mice. In: Biology of Radiation Carcinogenesis, J. M. Yukas, R. W. Tennant, and J. D. Regan (eds.), pp. 237-244, New York: Raven Press, 1976.

63. Lowy, D. R., Chattopadhyay, S. K., Teich, N. M., Rowe, W. P., and Levine, A. S., AKR murine leukemia virus genome: frequency of expression in DNA of high, low and non-virus yielding mouse strains, Proc. Natl. Acad. Sci., U.S.A., 71:3555-3559, (1974).

64. Lwoff, A., Lysogeny, Bacteriologic Reviews, 17:269-337, (1953).

65. Manteuil-Brutlag, S., Liu, S.-L., and Kaplan, H. S., Radiation leukemia virus contains two distinct viral RNAs, Cell, 19:643-652, (1980).

66. Mathieson, B. J., Campbell, P. S., Potter, M., and Asofsky, R., Expression of Ly 1, Ly 2, Thy 1, and TL differentiation antigens on mouse T-cell tumors, J. Exp. Med., 147:1267-1279, (1978).

67. McEndy, D. P., Boon, M. C., and Furth, J., On the role of thymus, spleen, and gonads in the development of leukemia in a high-leukemia stock of mice, Cancer Res., 4:377-383, (1944).

68. Nagao, K., Hamada, K., and Yokoro, K., Relationship between type-C RNA virus infectivity and leukemogenesis in N-nitrosomethylurea-treated NIH/Swiss mice, Proc. of the Japanese Cancer Ass'n., Tokyo, Japan, p. 283, 1978.

69. Nexo, B. J. and Ulrich, K., Activation of C-type virus during chemically induced leukemogenesis in mice, Cancer Res., 38:729-735, (1978).

70. Odaka, T., Strain-dependent expression of endogenous mouse-tropic leukemia viruses in chemically induced murine leukemias, Int. J. Cancer, 16:622-628, (1975).

71. Peters, R. L., Sass, B., Stephenson, J. R., Al-Ghazzouli, I. K., Hino, S., Donahoe, R. M., Kende, M., Aaronson, S. A., and Kelloff, G. J., Immunoprevention of x-ray-induced leukemias in the C57BL mouse, Proc. Natl. Acad. Sci., U.S.A., 74:1697-1701, (1977).

72. Philipson, L., Anderson, P., Olshevsky, U., Weinberg, R., Balti Baltimore, D., and Gesteland, R., Translation of MuLV and MSV RNAs in nuclease treated reticulocyte extracts: enhancement of

73. Ribacchi, R. and Giraldo, G., Leukemia virus release in chemically or physically induced lymphomas in BALB/c mice, *Natl. Cancer Inst. Monogr.*, *22:*701-711, (1966).

74. Riggin, C. H., Bondurant, M., and Mitchell, W. M., Physical properties of Moloney murine leukemia virus high molecular-weight RNA: a two subunit structure, *J. Virol.*, *16:*1528-1535, (1975).

75. Rothenberg, E., Donoghue, D. J., and Baltimore, D., Analysis of a 5' leader sequence on murine leukemia virus 21S RNA: heteroduplex mapping with long reverse transcriptase products, *Cell*, *13:*435-451, (1978).

76. Shields, A., Goff, S., Paskind, M., Otto, G., and Baltimore, D., Structure of the Abelson murine leukemia virus genome, *Cell, 18:* 955-962, (1979).

77. Simotohno, K., Mizutani, S., and Temin, H. M., Sequence of retrovirus provirus resembles that of bacterial transposable elements, *Nature, 285:*550-554, (1980).

78. Toth, B., Development of malignant lymphomas by cell-free filtrates from a chemically induced mouse lymphoma, *Proc. Soc. Exp. Biol. Med., 112:*873-875, (1963).

79. Upton, A. C., Jenkins, V. K., Walburg, H. E. Jr., Tyndall, R. L., Conklin, J. W., and Wald, N., Observations on viral, chemical, and radiation-induced myeloid and lymphoid leukemias in RF mice, *Natl. Cancer Inst. Monogr., 22:*329-345, (1966).

80. Vande Woude, G. F., Properties of two regions of the Moloney leukemia virus genome required for efficient transformation of src/sarc. In: Modern Trends in Leukemia IV, R. Neth and K. Mannweiler (eds.), Berlin: Springer-Verlag, in press.

81. Witte, O. N., Weissman, I. L., and Kaplan, H. S., Structural characteristics of some murine RNA tumor viruses studied by lactoperonidase iodination, *Proc. Natl. Acad. Sci., U.S.A., 70:*36-40, (1973).

—

RADIATION-INDUCED LEUKEMOGENESIS IN RFM/UN STRAIN MICE: A POTENTIAL MODEL FOR RETROVIRUS SEQUENCE TRANSPOSITION

Raymond W. Tennant[*]
Russell Earl Hand, Jr.
James A. Otten
Ruey-shyan Liou
J. O. Kiggans, Jr.
Wen K. Yang

Biology Division
Oak Ridge National Laboratory
Oak Ridge, Tennessee

Tse-Wei Wang

The University of Tennessee
Oak Ridge Graduate School of Biomedical Sciences
Oak Ridge, Tennessee

SUMMARY

The RFM/Un mouse strain is characterized by a significant life short-ening after a single dose of radiation, principally due to hematopoi-etic neoplasms. The strain is also unique in that there is a relative-ly high rate of myeloid leukemia which is induced following irradiation, and indirect evidence has implicated type C retroviruses as co-etio-logic agents. Analysis of various tissues from normal and tumor-bearing mice, including bone marrow, spleen, thymus, and embryonic cells, showed low-level expression of viral p 30 protein or an infec-tious type C virus. However, it was possible to cultivate and estab-lish cell lines from embryonic tissues and adult thymuses that were virus-negative but which could be chemically induced to express retro-virus. In all cases, only ecotropic virus with N-tropic host range was detected, and the production of a similar virus was detected in transplantable myeloid leukemia cells. Virus isolates of RFM/Un endo-genous origin showed good infectivity in most $Fv-1^n$ cells such as NIH Swiss mouse embryo cells but were severely restricted in $Fv-1^b$ cells, confirming the N-tropic host range; in addition, the replication of this RFM/Un endogenous N-tropic virus (RFV) was preferentially restrict-ed in RFM/Un cells which are of the $Fv-1^n$ genotype.

Current Affiliation: National Toxicology Program, National Institute of Environmental Health Sciences, Research Triangle Park, North Carolina

     The restriction of RFM/Un cells for RFV was analyzed at the stage
of viral DNA formation by means of a modified Hirt extraction procedure
and the electrophoresis/diazobenzyloxymethyl-paper transfer/molecular
hybridization method; it was found that synthesis of both linear and
covalently closed circular forms of viral DNA, either by RFV or by
WN1802B B-tropic virus, was markedly inhibited in RFM/Un cells relative to that of Gross virus. Analysis by restriction endonuclease
EcoR1 digestion demonstrated that nuclear DNA of RFM/Un cells contained
multiple copies of endogenous type C retroviral genes, including distinct retroviral sequences not found in NIH Swiss mouse cells which
never express endogenous ecotropic viruses.

     These results suggest that the RFM/Un mouse may possess only one
inducible ecotropic host-range class of inducible virus and a unique
gene, possibly an allele of the Fv-1 locus, which specifically restricts
endogenous virus. This model is therefore of potential value for genetic studies on the mechanism and etiological role of endogenous
retrovirus sequence transposition in radiation leukemogenesis since
viral gene transposition can be studied without the complications of
exogenous infection.

INTRODUCTION

The RFM mouse strain was derived by Jacob Furth, along with the AKR

strain in the 1930's [1]. Unlike the AKR, the RFM has a relatively

long median life span (635-712 days) and the principal types of neo-

plasia in untreated animals are reticulum cell sarcomas and lung ade-

nomas [2]. Upton and colleagues demonstrated a radiogenic myeloid

leukemia which occurred predominately in male mice after exposure to

single acute (300 rad) doses of X rays [3,4] whereas the thymus is

the principal target of radiation-induced neoplasms in most mouse

strains. This was of particular significance because myeloid leukemias

are known to occur in humans exposed to high-level, whole-body radia-

tion [5]. In addition, the pathological features of the RFM myeloid

leukemia closely resembles chronic granulocytic leukemia in man [4,6].

While evidence implicating a retrovirus in the etiology of the disease

was found [3], there has not been a detailed biological characteriza-

tion of the putative myeloid leukemia virus. We therefore initiated

a study of the expression of endogenous retrovirus in RFM/Un mice.

The results of these studies have shown a complex relationship involv-

ing host regulatory functions that make this strain a potentially unique

model to study retroviral and/or radiation tumorigenesis.

TABLE 1
Neoplasia in Irradiated and Control RFM/Un Strain Mice[a]

Neoplasm Type	Control Incidence[b] (%)		Irradiated (300 rads) Incidence (%)	
	Female	Male	Female	Male
Thymic lymphoma	13.4	6.6	52.4	26.9
Myeloid leukemia	.77	1.3	5.2	19.9
Reticulum cell sarcoma	42.3	51.7	23.2	34.1
Total	56.5	59.6	80.8	79.9
Orarian tumors	2.4		47.8	
Pituitary tumors	6.6		20.9	
Harderian gland tumors	1.2	1.2	16.2	14.8
Lung adenomas	30.2	31.5	37.1	40.8

[a]From [7], with permission.
[b]Age adjusted.

RESULTS

An extensive analysis of radiation leukemogenesis in RFM/Un mice was
reported by Ullrich and Storer [7]. Their results, a portion of which
are shown in Table 1, demonstrated that males are less sensitive to
induction of thymic lymphoma than females and showed a predominantly
linear dose response to radiation. However, males were more sensitive
than females to induction of myeloid leukemia showing an age-adjusted
incidence of approximately 20% at a single 300 rad dose of γ-radiation.
Both irradiated males and females showed a decrease in the incidence
of reticulum cell sarcomas. Radiation-induced thymomas in C57BL/6
strain mice have been etiologically linked to retrovirus induction
[8,9] and there is preliminary evidence of viral involvement in the
RFM/Un strain [3,10]. Therefore, we attempted to determine if retrovirus expression could be correlated with the radiation-induced leukemia pattern in RFM/Un mice.

TABLE 2
Analysis of RFM/Un Tissues[a]

	Thymus[b] Section (FA)	Co-Cultivation With[c]								Virus[d] Tropism	RIA (ng/ml)[e]					
		SC-1				Mink					Thy		Spl		Serum	
		Thy	Spl	BM	Other	Thy	Spl	BM	Other		gp70	p30	gp70	p30	gp70	p30
Weanling mice	+	+	+	+	+	-	-	-	-	N	443	952	1520	1568	410	<37
Young adult (6 months)	+	+	+	+	+	-	-	-	-	N						
Irradiated (6 months) (250R)	+	+	+	+	+	-	-	-	-	N						
Cultured embryo					-				-							
RFM/3T3					-				-							
+ IdUrd[f]					+				-	N						
Thymic epithelium					-				-							
+ IdUrd[f]					+				-	N						
Myeloid leukemia					+				-	N						
Thymoma	+				+				-	N						

[a]Thy, thymus; Spl, spleen; BM, bone marrow.
[b]Frozen sections (4-5 micron) of thymus tissue were acetone fixed to a slide and stained with fluorescein-conjugated anti-Moloney leukemia virus antisera [11].
[c]Tissues were removed from the animals, dispersed, and co-cultivated with indicator cells in the presence of 2μg/ml of polybrene. After three subcultures, supernant fluid was removed, filtered, and inoculated onto SC-1 and CCL-64 cells. Coverslips were examined after 48 hr for virus production by immunofluorescence.
[d]When virus was deteced in the SC-1 cells or the RFM/Un tissues, tropism was determined by innoculating Swiss mouse embryo (Fv-1[n]) or BALB/c (Fv-1[b]) cells, followed by XC plaque assay.
[e]20% suspensions (w/v) were made of the tissues, detergent disrupted, and clarified. The solubilized fraction was assayed by radioimmunoassay [13].
[f]Cells were treated with 50 μg/ml of IdUrd for 24 hr. The cultues were washed once and indicator cells were added in the presence of polybrene. Coverslips were harvested and assayed for virus protein by immunofluorescence.

Endogenous Retrovirus Expression

The results of our analysis of retrovirus expression in RFM/Un tissues, shown in Table 2, demonstrate that both virus proteins, detected by immunofluorescence assay [11] of thymus sections, and infectious virus detected by XC plaque assay [12] were present in hematopoietic tissues of both young and old, control and irradiated mice. In addition, radioimmunoassay [13] showed the presence of both gp70 and p30 proteins in spleens, thymus, and serum of weanling mice. However, cultured RFM/Un embryo cells did not express virus or virus protein and this may suggest the preferential expression of virus in hematopoietic cells. The secondary and tertiary RFM/Un embryo cells, as well as a line of RFM/3T3 cells that we derived, could be induced to express virus protein by growth for 24 hr in medium containing 50 μg/ml 5'-iododeoxyuridine (IdUrd). Virus was also detected in cultured thymoma and myeloid cells. However, adherent epithelial cells cultured from a spontaneous thymoma showed no detectable virus but could be induced to express virus protein by treatment with IdUrd. Both the cultured thymoma and myeloid cells grew as nonadherent populations and produced neoplasms of the respective histological type upon inoculation into either weanling RFM/Un mice or nude (athymic) nu/nu mice on an NIH Swiss background. Briefly, the principal pathologic features of thymic lymphoma in RFM/Un mice consist of a mediastinal mass and frequent infiltration of spleen, liver, and peripheral nodes with a uniform cell population resembling immature lymphocytes. The myeloid leukemia is of a granulocytic type which routinely involves the spleen and liver with frequent lymph node involvement, lung petechia, and bone marrow necrosis [14]. The transplantable tumor cells induced growth which closely resembled the primary disease patterns.

All virus isolates were characteristic of N-tropic murine retroviruses. We encountered difficulties in detecting virus isolated from cell-free material and, therefore, utilized co-cultivation with SC-1 mouse cells or CCL64 mink cells to amplify the virus production, which was then detectable with XC plaque and immunofluorescence assays. Virus was isolated only in SC-1 cells, and all isolates tested demonstrated preferential growth on NIH Swiss (Fv-1^n) over BALB/c (Fv-1^b) cells, confirming a clear N-tropism [15]. No virus of B-, xeno- or mixed-tropism was detected in any attempted isolations, using techniques (including co-cultivation with mink cells) which have been successful in demonstrating such viruses in cells from other mouse strains [16].

Analysis of Endogenous Virus Sequences

Previous work by Chattopadhyay et al. [17] revealed that the germ-line DNA of the mouse contains integrated copies of type C retroviral genes. Since IdUrd treatment can induce RFM/Un cells to produce N-tropic type C retrovirus this indicates that the genome of this particular virus is present in the DNA of RFM/Un cells. In an attempt to identify this particular viral genome, nuclear DNA was isolated from RFM/Un cells, digested with restriction endonuclease EcoR1, and analyzed by the agarose gel electrophoresis/Southern transfer/molecular hybridization method [18]. As a comparison, the analysis was performed in parallel with nuclear DNA of NIH Swiss mouse cells, which do not produce ecotropic type C viruses by IdUrd treatment and are known to contain only murine xenotropic type C viral genomes [19]. Preliminary results of the comparative analysis showed more complex patterns of viral DNA sequences in the RFM/Un cell DNA than in the NIH Swiss mouse cell DNA (Figure 1). Whether or not the inducible N-tropic virus locus corresponds to one of the distinct EcoR1-generated viral bands from RFM/Un nuclear DNA remains to be investigated.

Restriction of Endogenous Virus

Since the RFM/Un strain is of the Fv-1^n genotype [16] and the only host range type of virus detected in these cells was N-tropic, it would be expected that the virus could efficiently infect and spread in RFM/Un cells. However, it was very difficult to detect infectious virus in IdUrd-treated RFM/Un cells, even when up to 10% of the cells were induced to express virus protein. These results could represent

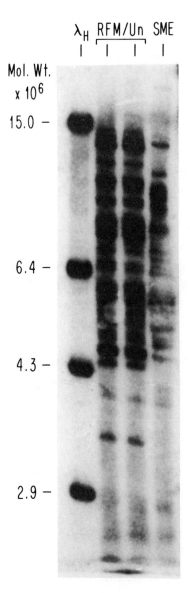

Figure 1. ECO-R1 restriction pattern of total nuclear DNA from SME and RFM/3T3 cells. Total DNA was extracted from nucleus preparations of confluent cell cultures and digested extensively with Eco-R1 endonuclease. Samples of 15-20 μg DNA were used for electrophoresis. The DNA was then denatured, neutralized, and transferred to nitrocellulose paper by the Southern procedure and analyzed by hybridization with ^{32}P-cDNA prepared from genomic RNA of WN1802B ecotropic virus. Autoradiography was performed with Kodak X-O-matic X-ray film and intensifying screens at -70°C for 4 days. The markers used were Hind-III fragments of bacteriophage lambda DNA.

differential induction of viral protein synthesis, induction of non-
infectious virus, or an inability of infectious virus to spread to
other RFM/Un cells and establish productive infection. A comparison
was made of the titration patterns of the endogenous RFM/Un virus
(RFV), isolated by co-cultivation with SC-1 cells and three other viruses (WN1802N, an endogenousN-tropic virus from BALB/c mice; AKR,
an endogenous N-tropic virus of the AKR strain; and Gross leukemia
virus (GLV), a leukemogenic virus originally derived from C3H mice)
in six cell strains (Table 3).

   All four viruses infected SC-1 (Fv-1$^-$) cells to a comparable high
degree and were highly restricted in BALB/3T3 (Clone A31) (Fv-1^b) cells
with discrete two-hit kinetics, consistent with N-tropism. However,
while RFV infected C3H, AKR, and NIH/3T3 (all Fv-1^n) cells to a comparable degree, it was restricted greater than three logs in RFM/Un
cells so that no titer could be determined. In addition, the XN1802N
and AKR viruses also demonstrated a significant restriction in the
RFM/Un cells with two-hit kinetics. In contrast, there was only about
a one-log restriction of GLV, which demonstrated single-hit kinetics.
These results demonstrate a significant restriction of RFM/Un cells
for endogenous viruses, particularly the virus derived from RFM/Un
cells, relative to that for exogenous Gross virus.

TABLE 3

Titration Patterns of Virus Stocks on Cells of Different Fv-1 Genotypes

Cell	Fv-1 Genotype	Titer $(\log_{10})^a$			
		WN1802N	RFV	AKR	GLV
C3H	nn	4.4×10^5	3.9×10^2	2.8×10^5	ND
RFM/3T3	nn	1.3×10^2	$10'$	4.6×10^2	1.4×10^5
AKR	nn	9.4×10^4	2.9×10^2	8.3×10^4	2.1×10^6
NIH/3T3	nn	5.4×10^5	2.6×10^2	7.1×10^5	6.0×10^6
BALB/3T3 (Clone A31)	bb	7.2×10^2	$10'$	1.5×10^4	5.0×10^3
SC1	--	8.3×10^6	8.7×10^3	3.3×10^6	2.0×10^6

[a]The cells were plated in 35-mm wells and 18 hr later the media was removed and the cells treated with DEAE-dextran (25 µg/ml) for 30 min.
DEAE was removed, and the cells were washed and then infected with virus
for 1 hr. The virus was removed and 5 days later XC plaque titrations
were performed.

Restriction Mechanisms

A major effort of our laboratory has been to study the mechanism of
restriction of murine retroviruses by the mouse Fv-1 locus. A key
aspect of these studies has been the kinetic analysis of viral DNA
formation, via reverse transcription, in the early phase of infection
(0-12 hr) and a measurement of the linear (form III) and circular forms
(I and II) of viral DNAs in Fv-1 restrictive and permissive cells.
Viral DNA was extracted using a modified Hirt [20] procedure and the
gel electrophoresis/diazobenzyloxymethyl-paper transfer/molecular hybridization method [21]. The major finding was that the appearance
of the two species of covalently closed circular DNAs was quantitative-
ly depressed in Fv-1 restrictive cells according to the two-hit pattern
of virus-dose response. Specifically, the number of circular DNAs
of GLV (N-tropic) detected in BALB/c cells (Fv-1^b) was proportional
to the square of the dose of virus infecting the cells, whereas the
number of linear DNA duplex molecules formed by the same virus in permissive (Fv-1^n) cells was directly proportional to the amount of virus
inoculated [21]. These results and those of others [22] support the
hypothesis that the covalently closed circular supercoiled form I of
retroviral DNA is an obligatory intermediate, presumably for gene integration, in the replication cycle of retroviruses, and that the primary function of the Fv-1 locus is to restrict the formation of this
intermediate form of viral DNA.

In this study, using the same technical approach, we found a distinctive feature of Fv-1 restriction in RFM/Un mouse embryo cells relative to NIH Swiss cells (Figure 2). Unlike some other Fv-1^n (DBA/2)
and most Fv-1^b cells examined, the RFM/Un and NIH Swiss cells showed
a marked inhibition of the formation of linear duplex DNA by B-tropic
(WN1802B) virus. In addition, the linear duplex DNA formation by the
RFV virus was preferentially inhibited in RFM/Un cells (Figure 3).
These results indicate that the RFM/Un cells may possess a more restrictive allele of the Fv-1^n gene for B-tropic virus and also a significant restriction of endogenous N-tropic virus infection reflected
in the depressed formation of linear duplex viral DNA. The possible
relationship of RFV virus restriction in RFM/Un cells to the Fv-1
locus remains to be defined.

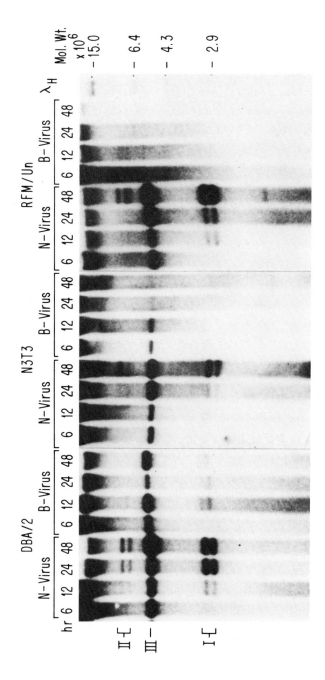

Figure 2. Autoradiograms showing formation of viral DNA intermediates in Fv-1^n mouse cells. The cells were inoculated with Gross N-tropic (Nv) or WN1802B B-tropic (Bv) virus at an m.o.i. of 0.5 and examined for viral DNAs 6, 12, 24, and 48 hr after virus inoculation [20]. I, covalently closed circular supercoiled forms; II, open circular forms; III, linear forms.

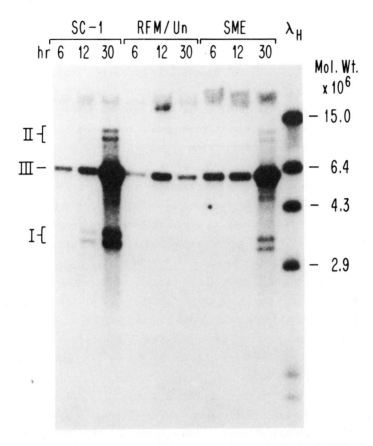

Figure 3. Autoradiogram showing synthesis of RFV viral DNAs in SC-1 cells, RFM/3T3 cells and NIH Swiss mouse embryo (SME) cells. At 6, 12, and 30 hours after RFV inoculation at an m.o.i. of 0.5, the cells were extracted for unintegrated viral DNAs with a modified Hirt extraction procedure. DNA preparations were separated by electrophoresis in 0.6% agarose gel, transferred to diazobenzyloxymethyl-paper and hybridized with [^{32}P]-labeled viral copy DNA. Positions of linear duplex form (III), closed circular supercoiled duplex forms (I) and open circular duplex forms (II) of viral DNA were indicated. Hind III generated λ phage DNA fragments served as molecular weight markers for linear DNA duplexes. Each lane represents DNA samples from cells in one 100 mm dish (1.58 x 10^6 SC-1 cells, 1.73 x 10^6 RFM/3T3 cells and 1.66 x 10^6 SME cells at the time of infection; cell growth was comparable in the 30 hr post infection period). Autoradiography was carried out for 15 hours.

DISCUSSION

The etiological role of retroviruses in radiation leukogenesis has
been extensively analyzed in C57BL/6 strain mice [8]. At least three
distinct host range types of virus have been isolated from both normal
cells and radiation-induced tumors, and a new class of B-tropic virus,
which preferentially infects thymocytes (thymotropic virus), was defined [23]. The characteristics of this thymotropic agent strongly
suggest an etiological role in radiation-induced thymic lymphoma [9].
Unlike the C57BL/6 strain, we have been able to demonstrate only one
(N-tropic) host-range class of virus in both normal and tumor cells
of RFM/Un mice. This virus is expressed at low levels in hematopoietic
tissues throughout the life-span of RFM/Un mice. No measurable increase in expression is associated with irradiation, and the virus
exhibits no unusual cellular tropism. These results indicate that in
the RFM/Un strain radiation-induced leukemogenesis may involve some
mechanisms of induction or pathogenesis different from that of the
C57BL strain. While the two alleles of the FV-1 locus (n and b) have
been well defined, Pincus [16] found evidence of another type of allele called nr. Cells from strains NZB, NZW, 129 and RF/J showed a
significantly lower sensitivity to N-tropic virus relative to the pro-
totype $Fv-1^n$ NIH Swiss strain. Other evidence that the RF/J strain
possessed a degree of resistance to N-tropic virus relative to the AKR
strain was seen by Pincus et al. [24]. Subsequently Mayer et al. [25]
studied the frequency of lymphoma development in F_1 hybrids of AKR/J
and RF/J mice and found that hybrids developed the disease at a lower
frequency and later in life than the AKR parent (but at a somewhat
higher rate than the RF/J parent). Backcross-mating indicated involvement of a single dominant gene and studies utilizing glucose-6-
phosphate dehydrogenase ($Gpd-1^a$) as a linkage marker demonstrated that
lymphoma resistance segregated with the RF/J allele of the Fv-1 locus.
The reduced expression of virus in F_1 generation mice and the segrega-
tion of this dominant suppression with the $Gdp-1^a$ allele of the RF/J
parent in an AKR x (AKR x RF) backcross also directly implicates the

Fv-1 locus. Subsequent studies provided evidence of a maternal-specif-
ic suppression of lymphoma which appeared to be independent of, but
additive to, the Fv-1 effect [26]. Thus, the combination of a limited
host range class of endogenous virus together with a restriction specific for the virus qualifies the RFM/Un strain as a unique system
in which to study radiation leukemogenesis.

If the virus is etiologically involved in hematopoietic neoplasia,
spontaneous or radiation-induced, in this strain then intercellular
spread may be a key element in the process. While virus expression
appears to be prevalent in hematopoietic cells, infectious virus is
relatively difficult to detect, suggesting incomplete virus synthesis
or that released virus has a reduced infectivity, even for cells which
lack the RFM-type restriction. The relatively late-life spontaneous
rate of hematopoietic neoplasia may be a reflection of the low-level
virus infectivity together with the unique restriction of RFM/Un cells
for this virus. The effect of radiation in increasing the frequency
of myeloid leukemia and thymic lymphoma could involve an indirect effect of stimulating the proliferation of stem cells which express viral
genes, and irradiation might serve to increase the probability that
a virus-positive stem cell is stimulated to divide as a result of
cellular depletion.

In the case of the myeloid leukemias, characteristics of the pathogenesis and properties of the neoplastic cells suggest an alteration
of cellular differentiation, probably involving specific hematopoietic
stem cells [6]. This pattern suggests a block in the differentiation
pattern of certain granulocytic cells, somewhat similar to the pattern
seen in the erythrocytic leukemia induced by Friend leukemia virus
[27,28] in which spread of the virus is not restricted.

Recent studies on the fine structure of the retrovirus genome
suggest a new mechanism for retrovirus involvement in the heritable
alteration of stem cell differentiation. It has been established in
both prokaryotic and eukaryotic systems that certain gene elements
are capable of transposition from one genetic locus to another. These
elements, called transposons, can cause rapid changes in an organism
such as antiobiotic resistance in bacteria, mating types in yeast,

and inheritance of traits not predictable by Mendelian laws or linkage
maps in maize [29]. Although being completely heterogeneous in nucleotide sequence composition, the fine structure of all transposons show
unique physical characteristics in that stretches of exact repeat sequences (in a direct and/or inverted manner) are present on both ends
of the linear DNA molecule. Experimental evidence suggests that these
DNA repeats play a key role in the mechanism of transposition. Recent
evidence [30,31] has established that retroviral DNAs contain unique
structural features similar to those of prokaryotic transposons and
that in the well studied cases of chickens and mice the genome of
retroviruses is detected in multiple copies in the chromatin DNA of
the cell (and are called endogenous retroviral genes) [16]. While
these retroviral genes are usually inherited in a Mendelian fashion,
they have a demonstrated capacity to be induced when cellular DNA metabolism is perturbed [32]. For example, treatment of cultured mouse
cells with IdUrd, hydroxyurea, X-irradiation or some chemical carcinogens, induces the cells to produce "type C" viruses [32]. Thus it
appears that the endogenous retroviral genes initiate a transposition
mechanism by transcription into genomic RNA (infectious virus). In
the process of horizontal infection and subsequent integration into
new genetic loci, the RNA genome of the virus is reversely transcribed
into a DNA molecule containing the terminal repeat DNA sequences of
a transposon.

In the course of gene transpositions, the genome of retroviruses
may recombine (and hence incorporate) other cellular gene sequences
into its transposon structure. Once incorporated, the normal cellular
gene sequence may become abnormal in that it is now capable of insert-
ing into a different genetic locus within the cell and become subject
to very different regulatory mechanisms or control of gene expression.
Actually, all oncogenic retrovirus genes responsible for inducing neoplastic transformation in the cell have been found to be of cellular
origin [33]. In this regard the "oncogene" is therefore a normal cellular structural gene linked to "insertion gene sequences." In this
view, retroviral genes are related to carcinogenesis not directly but
indirectly through genetic mechanisms of gene transposition. An

exogenous carcinogen such as radiation may act either by inducing an
endogenous retroviral gene sequence, by enhancing a recombinational
event, or by promoting the metabolic process for production of oncogene
precursors. All of these possibilities can be experimentally determined since utilization of molecular probes (specific copy DNA of
retroviral genes) can now be developed.

The RFM/Un strain mouse, therefore, provides a relatively unique
approach to the problem of transposition of retroviral sequences since
it appears that changes in the virus locus essentially can occur only
through intragenomic transposition. The transposition would be per-
petuated by proliferation of daughter cells in which the transposition
occurred. If such transpositions are limited to a finite number of
loci and if such a locus (or loci) exists within the transcriptional
domain of hematopoietic differentiation, it is possible that terminal
differentiation of stem cells could be heritably altered, thus leading
to a leukemic state. Since cell clones of myeloid leukemias induced
by irradiation of RFM/Un mice can be isolated for molecular study,
this hypothesis will be subjected to vigorous tests in our laboratories.

ACKNOWLEDGMENTS

This research was sponsored jointly by the National Cancer Institute
under Interagency Agreement Y01 CP 60500 and the Office of Health and
Environmental Research U.S. Department of Energy, under contract
W-7405-eng-26 with the Union Carbide Corporation.

Dr. Wang and Dr. Liou are Postdoctoral Investigators supported
by subcontract 3322 from the Biology Division of Oak Ridge National
Laboratory to the University of Tennessee.

The authors gratefully acknowledge the thoughtful discussions
and critique of this work by Stephen J. Kennel and Arthur Brown.

REFERENCES

1. Furth, J., Seibold, H. R., and Rathbone, R. R., *Am. J. Cancer*, *19*:521-604 (1933).

2. Clapp, N. K., Darden, E. B., and Jernigan, M. C., *Radiat. Res.*, *57*:158-186 (1974).

3. Jenkins, V. K., and Upton, A. C., *Cancer Res.*, *23*:1748-1755 (1963).

4. Upton, A. C., Jenkins, V. K., and Conklin, J. W., *Ann. N. Y. Acad. Sci.*, *114*:189-201 (1964).

5. Brill, A. B., Tomanaga, M., and Heyssel, R. M., *Ann. Intern. Med.*, *56*:590-609 (1962).

6. Fialkow, P. J., Gartler, S. M., and Yoshida, A., *Proc. Natl. Acad. Sci., U.S.A.*, *58*:1468-1471 (1967).

7. Ullrich, R. L., and Storer, J. B., *Radiat. Res.*, *80*:303-316 (1979).

8. Kaplan, H. S., Interaction between radiation and viruses in the induction of murine thymic lymphomas and lymphatic leukemias. In: Radiation-Induced Leukemogenesis and Related Viruses (J. F. Duplan, ed.), North Holland Publishing Co., Amsterdam, 1977, pp. 1-18.

9. Kaplan, H. S., These proceedings, 1981.

10. Tanako, T., and Craig, A. W., *Eur. J. Cancer, 6*:329-333 (1970).

11. Hand, R. E. Jr., Tennant, R. W., Yang, W. K., and Lavelle, G., *J. Immunol. Methods, 23*:175-186 (1978).

12. Rowe, W. P., Pugh, W. P., and Hartley, J. W., *Virology, 42*:1136-1139 (1970).

13. Kennel, S. J., and Tennant, R. W., *J. Virol., 30*:729-734 (1979).

14. Clapp, N. K., An Atlas of RF Mouse Pathology: Disease Descriptions and Incidences. USAEC Technical Information Center Publication TID 26373, U.S. Dept. of Commerce, Springfield, VA, 1973.

15. Jolicoeur, P., *Curr. Top. Microbiol. Immunol., 86*:68-122 (1980).

16. Pincus, T., The endogenous murine type C viruses. In: Molecular Biology of RNA Tumor Viruses (John R. Stephenson, ed.), Academic Press, 1980, pp. 77-130.

17. Chattopadhyay, S. K., Lowy, D. R., Teich, N. M., Levine, A. S., and Rowe, W. P., *Cold Spring Harbor Symp. Quant. Biol., 39*:1085-1101 (1974).

18. Southern, E. M., *J. Mol. Biol., 98:*503-517 (1975).

19. Rowe, W. P., Leukemia virus genomes in the chromosomal DNA of the mouse. Harvey Lectures 1975-1976, Academic Press, 1978, pp. 173-192.

20. Hirt, B., *J. Mol. Biol., 26:*365-369 (1967).

21. Yang, W. K., Kiggans, J. O., Yang, D.-M., Ou, C.-Y., Tennant, R. W., Brown, A., and Bassin, R. H., *Proc. Natl. Acad. Sci., U.S.A., 77:*2994-2998 (1980).

22. Jolicoeur, P., and Rassart, E., *J. Virol., 33:*183-195 (1980).

23. Decleve, A., Sato, C., Lieberman, M., and Kaplan, H. S., *Proc. Natl. Acad. Sci., U.S.A., 71:*3124-3128 (1974).

24. Pincus, T., Hartley, J. W., and Rowe, W. P., *J. Exp. Med., 133:*1219-1233 (1971).

25. Mayer, A., Duran-Reynals, M. L., and Lilly, F., *Cell, 15:*429-435 (1978).

26. Mayer, A., Struuck, F. D., Duran-Reynals, M. L., and Lilly, F., *Cell, 19:*431-435 (1980).

27. Friend, C., Scher, W., Tsuei, D., Haddad, J., Holland, J. G., Szrajer, N., and Haubenstock, H., Perspectives on Friend leukemia virus: Pathogenesis in vivo and studies on the control of erythro differentiation in vitro in oncogenic viruses and host cell genes. In: Oncogenic Viruses and Host Cell Genes (Y. Ikawa and T. Odaka, eds.), Academic Press, 1979, pp. 279-299.

28. Marks, P. A., and Rifkind, R. A., *Annu. Rev. Biochem., 47:*419-448 (1978).

29. Calos, M. P., and Miller, J. H., *Cell, 20:*579-595 (1980).

30. Taylor, J. M., Mason, W. S., Hsu, T. W., Sabran, J. L., Yeater, C., Mark, G. E., Kaji, A., Guntaka, R. V., and Lai, M. M. C., *Cold Spring Harbor Symp. Quant. Biol., 43:*865-867 (1979).

31. Hughes, S. H., Shank, P. R., Specta, D. H., Kung, H.-J., Bishop, J. M., and Varmus, H. E., *Cell, 15:*1397-1410 (1978).

32. Tennant, R. W., and Rascati, R. J., Mechanisms of cocarcinogenesis involving endogenous retroviruses. In: Carcinogenesis, Vol. 5, T. J. Slaga, ed.), Raven Press, New York, 1980, pp. 185-206.

33. Wang, L. H., Snyder, P., Hanafusa, T., and Hanafusa, H., *J. Virol., 35:*52-64 (1980).

MECHANISM OF NEOPLASTIC TRANSFORMATION OF CULTURED MAMMALIAN CELLS BY HERPES SIMPLEX VIRUS TYPE 2 OR CHEMICAL CARCINOGENS: A UNIFIED HYPOTHESIS

Laure Aurelian

Department of Biochemistry and Biophysics
The Johns Hopkins Medical Institutions
Baltimore, Maryland

Mark M. Manak

Departments of Biophysics and Comparative Medicine
The Johns Hopkins Medical Institutions
Baltimore, Maryland

Paul O. P. Ts'o

Division of Biophysics
School of Hygiene and Public Health
The Johns Hopkins Medical Institutions
Baltimore, Maryland

PROGRAM

Cancer, one of the most dreaded diseases of our time, originated from a single cell, or a group of cells, that have escaped regulatory controls and have achieved immortality by the multi-step acquisition of an unlimited ability to replicate. Squamous carcinoma of the human cervix, the second most prevalent cancer in human females, is a paradigm of the multi-step, progressive aspect of human neoplasia. Thus, invasive cancer is preceded by pre-neoplastic lesions designated dysplasia and carcinoma in situ (CIS), a proportion of which (20-40%) will progress to frank neoplasia [1].

Consistent with its infectious (sexual) transmission pattern, cervix cancer has been associated with the sexually transmitted herpesvirus type 2 (HSV-2) on the basis of multidisciplinaty evidence recently reviewed by Rawls and Adam [2], and by Aurelian et al. [3].

229

TABLE 1
HSV-2 and Cervix Cancer

1. Infection with HSV-2 more common in cancer cases than in controls.

2. Cancer incidence 4-16 fold higher in women with herpetic cervicitis than in uninfected controls.

3. HSV-2 infection precedes the earliest pre-neoplastic lesion. Pre-neoplastic lesions progress to invasive cancer.

4. Association of HSV-2 with cervix cancer shows immunologic specificity.

5. Specific virus genes are continuously expressed in cervix cancer cases but not in controls. Tumor cells are positive for antigens/proteins AG-4, AG-e, and VP134.

6. Tumor cells are positive for virus-specific mRNA[a].

7. Viral DNA sequences reported in invasive cancer. Distinct HSV-2 strain isolated from pre-neoplastic lesion.

8. HSV-2 induces tumorigenic transformation. Transformed cells express viral antigens.

9. Animal model: HSV-2 infected Cebus monkeys develop preneoplastic lesions.

[a]From [4].
Source: Adapted from [2] and [3].

Briefly (Table 1), infection with HSV-2 is more prevalent in women with cervix cancer than in normal control women matched for other disease-associated variables. The relative risk of cancer in women with herpetic cervicitis is 4-16 fold higher than in women without similar herpetic disease and infection with HSV-2 precedes by a mean of 6 years the development of the earliest detectable lesions (dysplasia). Viral antigens, designated AG-e, VP134, and AG-4, are expressed in cervical tumor cells. Cervix cancer patients display specific humoral (VP134 and AG-4) and/or cell-mediated immune (AG-e) responses against these viral proteins. At least one of them (AG-4) reflects the progression of the cervical tumor. It is associated

TABLE 2
ICP 10: A Hypothetical HSV-2 vtr[a]

---

1. Phosphorylated viral protein, 161,000 daltons.

2. "Early" onset of synthesis (2 hours p.i.) in productive in-
    fection. Maximal levels 4-9 hours p.i.

3. Immediate "early" protein: Synthesis does not require previ-
    ous viral protein synthesis.

4. Primary cellular location: Cytoplasm and nuclear membrane.
    Also located on cell surface.

5. Expressed in cells neoplastically transformed by viral DNA
    sequences spanning map coordinates 43-58.

6. Expression strongly correlated with anchorage independence
    and tumorigenicity.

7. Immunologically identical to antigen AG-4 expressed in human
    cervical cells and reflecting the progression of the cervical
    tumor.

---

[a]Postulated vtr (viral transforming protein) is encoded by the
transforming viral DNA sequences (VTR) and is associated with the
maintenance of a transformed phenotype (Figure 4).

with 35-45% of pre-neoplastic and 86% of invasive lesions. AG-4 is
immunologically identical to ICP 10 (Table 2), a phosphorylated, "immediate early", infected cell protein (ICP), that in productively infected cells accumulates at the nuclear membrane. Viral DNA sequences
were reported in a cervical tumor, a distinct HSV-2 strain (differs
from laboratory strains in DNA restriction endonuclease cleavage pattern) was isolated from cultured cells established from a CIS biopsy,
and virus-specific RNA was observed in cervical tumor cells by in situ
hybridization [4]. Finally, inactivated HSV-2 or high dilutions of
native non-inactivated HSV-2 DNA transform cultured mammalian cells
to a neoplastic phenotype and consistent with the human observations,
35% of Cebus monkeys infected vaginally with HSV-2 develop non-regres-
sive cervical dysplasia within 5 years post infection.

    We have previously suggested [5] that if HSV-2 plays an etiologic
role in cervical cancer, it most probably acts as an <u>initiator</u> in the

progression of normal to tumorigenic cells. This interpretation argues
that in vivo HSV-2 induced phenotypic alterations destined to progress
to cervix cancer (dysplasia), are analogous to the neoplastic transformation of cultured cells. Accordingly, our recent studies have
focused on the neoplastic potential of HSV-2, using the in vitro transformation of mammalian (Syrian hamster embryo, SHE) cells as a model
system. The experimental design posited neoplastic potential as the
only viable criterion for transformation, thus establishing HSV-2 as
a complete carcinogen. However, consistent with the hypothesis that
HSV-2 acts as an initiator, two cell lines were established in the
course of these studies that although non-tumorigenic had achieved
immortality and acquired the ability to grow in low serum. Similar
results were independently obtained in other cell systems transformed
with HSV-2 ([6]; Kucera, personal communication).

The consistent end-point of the transforming event (immortality
and invasion stands in absolute contradistinction to the diversity of
the carcinogens capable of inducing it. The data and interpretations
discussed in this presentation will reflect the premise that the consistent outcome of transformation by different carcinogens is due to
the fact that at the molecular level this outcome is, at least in part,
under cellular control. Although we will focus on transformation by
HSV-2 and by direct perturbation to host cell DNA, presently available
data will be discussed within the context of our beliefs that: (i)
the mechanism(s) of regulation/differentiation, (ii) the programming
of gene expression and (iii) the progression of de-regulated cells
to their ultimate conclusion (i.e., immortality or senescence) are
the major problems in carcinogenesis at the present time.

Transformation of Syrian Hamster Embryo (SHE) Fibroblasts by DNA Perturbation

Consideration of those perturbations that delineate critical target
molecules inside the cells seems particularly profitable. Such perturbations to DNA alone were extensively studies in one of our laboratories with tumorigenic potential as the ultimate endpoint. As
recently reviewed by Ts'o [7], these studies were designed to address

the following questions: (i) what effect will a specific attack on
DNA have on neoplastic transformation, (ii) what, if any, is the relationship between neoplastic transformation and mutation, (iii) is
there a relationship between neoplasia and an in vitro acquired altered
phenotype and (iv) what is the mechanism for the acquisition of these
altered growth characteristics.

Analysis of benzo(a)pyrene [B(a)P] transformed SHE clonal lines
that differed in tumorigenic potential and in in vitro growth properties, revealed that anchorage independent growth (cloning in 0.3% agar
or agarose) was highly correlated (99% confidence level, $p \leq 0.01$ according to Kendall's coefficient of rank correlation) with tumorigenicity. Although significant (95% confidence level, $p \leq 0.05$), fibrinolytic activity and growth in low serum (1%) appeared to represent weak-
er correlates of tumorigenic potential [8]. Unlike somatic mutation
[9], the neoplastic transformation process appeared to be progressive
in nature rather than a single-step phenomenon. Thus, morphological
changes and enhanced fibrinolytic activity were observed early after
treatment with B(a)P, whereas the ability to grow in semisolid agar
was delayed to 32-75 population doublings post exposure to carcinogen.
A large percentage of cells isolated at early passage expressed anchorage independent growth only after their independent in vitro passage
to at least 32 population doublings (pd), indicating that neoplastic
transformation in vitro is a progressive process through qualitatively
different stages.

Direct perturbation of DNA was accomplished by a number of procedures. One such procedure [10] involved the incorporation of BUdR
into DNA in place of its analog thymidine. Since the UV adsorption
spectrum is thus shifted towards a larger wavelength, the irradiation
of this substituted DNA with light of wavelengths greater than 300 nm
(near UV light) produces a significantly higher number of photochemical
lesions that are produced in unsubstituted DNA. These lesions are
mostly single-strand breaks caused by an initial photodissociation of
the bromine atom producing uracylil radical that is then decomposed.
When cells in different stages of their growth cycle were treated for
1 hour with BUdR and then irradiated with near (nUV) light, it was
found that morphologic transformation occurred with maximal frequency

when treatment was done in middle of S (DNA synthesis period) phase.
Growth in agar and tumorigenicity were observed in these cells after
100-150 days in culture.

Specific nuclear DNA damage due to incorporation of methyl ^{3}H-
thymidine also induced transformation. Morphologic alterations were
first seen at pd 3-4, subpopulations with increased fibrinolytic activity at pd 11-16, those capable of growing in 1% serum at pd 18-32
and those capable of growth in soft agar at pd 25-32. Tumorigenicity
was observed in all treated cells at pd 50. Finally, neoplastic transformation was observed in diploid SHE cells after treatment with lipo-
somes that contained DNase I [7].

Somatic mutation and neoplastic transformation were examined con-
comittantly. Mutations induced by B(a)P were quantitated at the HCPRT
locus (a sex-linked recessive mutation) and NA$^+$/K$^+$ ATPase locus (an
autosomal dominant or co-dominant mutation) and compared to morphologic
alteration and anchorage independence. Both of the transformation-
associated properties had characteristics different from those of
somatic mutation at the two studied loci. Morphologic transformation
was observed at a time comparable to somatic mutations but at a frequency 25-540 fold higher. Anchorage independence was found at a frequency (10^{-5} to 10^{-6}) similar to that of somatic mutations but not
until ptp 32-75 as compared to ptp 6-8 for somatic mutation [7,9].
Therefore, the data suggest that neoplastic transformation can be initiated by direct perturbation (viz. the generation of single strand
breaks) to DNA. However, transformation is more complex than a single-
gene mutational process, and it may involve the induction of an inter-
locked cascading set of events that will irrevocably commit the cells
to unregulated cell division.

HSV-2 Induced Transformation

In the absence of non-permissive in vitro systems, HSV-2 induced transformation was originally established with virus whose lytic functions
were inactivated [11-13]. Selection was based on: (i) morphologic
and growth alterations including, in some cases, neoplastic potential

[11-13], or (ii) the transfer of the HSV encoded thymidine kinase
(tk) gene to mouse cells previously lacking this function [14]. From
the standpoint of a unified hypothesis for the mechanism of transformation, the following problems merit further scrutiny: (i) is the maintenance of a transformed phenotype a function of the persistance/
expression of specific viral gene(s), and (ii) is neoplastic potential
acquired by a progressive, cell-determined, process through qualitatively different stages?

"Hit and run" hypothesis. The "hit and run" hypothesis argues that
continued viral gene expression is not required for the maintenance
of a transformed phenotype. It has gained a measure of support from
the observations that: (i) hamster embryo cells morphologically transformed [15] by a 15 x 10^6 daltons fragment of HSV-1 DNA (spanning map
units 20-45) are negative for HSV DNA sequences in relatively early
(< 15) passages [16], and (ii) murine cells morphologically transformed
by inactivated HSV-2 are negative for viral markers [17].

The experimental design of studies done in our laboratories on
this topic was based on the assumption that, according to the "hit
and run" hypothesis, transformation requires the one-time expression
of transforming viral function(s) encoded by the incoming parental
viral genome. Accordingly, expression of these functions, followed
by fragmentation of the incoming viral genome, should give rise at a
relatively high frequency, to transformed cells devoid of persistent
viral genetic information. The method that we selected in order to
test the validity of this interpretation consisted in the fragmentation
(and by inference the inactivation) of BUdR-substituted viral DNA at
various times during a synchronized replicative cycle, i.e. after the
expression of various viral functions had been completed.

HSV-2 (ANG) grown in presence of 10 μM BUdR (11% substitution
of thymidine residues) fulfilled the experimental requirements. It
retained virtually all its infectivity and displayed relatively high
levels (2 logs) of inactivation by nUV irradiation. The viral replicative cycle was synchronized by infection at relatively high m.o.i.
(5 PFU/cell) and any residual infectivity (1 in 10^3 PFU), probably

due to the presence of unsubstituted or minimally substituted DNA
molecules, was excluded by extinction dilution techniques. Consistent
with the finding that viral DNA synthesis (resulting progeny molecules
that are not BUdR-substituted and therefore are insensitive to nUV)
begins at 4 hours p.i. and reaches maximal levels by 8 hours, exposure
of BUdR-HSV-2 (ANG) infected cells to nUV at various times after infection, resulted in maximal inactivation of viral infectivity at 0-6
hours p.i., and was no longer possible by 10 hours p.i. HSV-2 induced
transformation occurred with maximal frequency when virus infectivity
was inactivated at 4 hours p.i. and did not increase at 6 or 8 hours
p.i. Two procedures were used to assay for transformation. One of
these, the focus-formation assay, is a quantitative procedure adapted
in our laboratory in medium containing 1% serum, a condition under
which normal SHE cells do not grow [18]. Under these conditions, morphologically altered colonies were observed in the virus-treated but
not in the normal SHE cells. However, in our hands, less than 10%
of isolated colonies were capable of growing into stable transformed
lines. Therefore, the significance of the assay with respect to carcinogenesis remains elusive. The second transformation assay used
in these studies was the continuous passage assay performed as described [19]. By comparison to the focus formation assay in 1% serum,
the frequency of transformation estimated by the continuous passage
procedure represents a lower limit figure, since even if multiple
transformation events occurred within a single plate, they were still
scored as one. Nevertheless, the two assays agreed in: (i) establishing the interval at which transformation occurs with maximal frequency
as 4-8 hours p.i., and (ii) demonstrating that the frequency of transformation is virtually identical in cells irradiated at 4, 6, and 8
hours p.i. As previously demonstrated [10], spontaneous transformation
was not observed in cells exposed to nUV light in absence of HSV-2
(Table 3).

    Transformed cells displayed morphologic and growth alterations,
were tumorigenic in newborn hamsters, and expressed viral antigens
(even at relatively late passage) as evidenced by their reactivity
(Table 4) with the IgG fraction of antisera to total viral proteins

TABLE 3

Frequency of Transformation by Virus Inactivated at Various Times in the Course of Productive Infection[a]

Time of inactivation	Preinac.	0 hrs	2 hr.	4 hr.	6 hrs.	8 hr.	10 hr.	Uninfected[d]
Focus formation/low serum Frequency[b]	0.5%	0.5%	0.75%	11.8%	7.5%	8.5%	CPE	0
Continuous passage Frequency[c]	<0.1%	<0.1%	<0.1%	0.38%	0.25%	0.33%	CPE	0

[a]SHE cells in suspension culture were exposed to 5 PFU/cell of BUdR-labeled HSV. Following adsorption, 100 cells were seeded with 10^5 uninfected cells, and exposed to nUV irradiation at the times indicated. CPE was observed when 10^4 infected cells were seeded under similar conditions.

[b]Frequency of transformation expressed as no. of foci/no. of treated cells.

[c]Frequency of transformation expressed as no. of lines/no. of treated cells.

[d]Twelve plates were exposed to nUV light in absence of HSV-2.

TABLE 4

Properties of SHE Cells Transformed by HSV-2 Inactivated at Various Times Post Infection[a]

Characteristic	SHE Passage 4	HBU-1 PTP 35	HT4A PTP 22	HT4A PTP 41	HT6A PTP 54	HT8A PTP 36
Predominant morphology	Fibroblast	Epitheloid	Epitheloid	Epitheloid	Fibroblast	Fibroblast
Saturation density (x 10^6 cells/cm^2)	1.2	3.9	4.6	3.4	4.2	4.7
Growth in 2% serum[b]	0	12.5	25	20	10	37
Anchorage independence[c]	0	2.9	1.8	10.0	6.2	23.6
Tumorigenicity[d]	0/12 (0)	2/6 (33)	3/6 (50)	8/11 (72)	2/6 (33)	4/7 (57)
Latent period	-	13 wks.	22 wks.	13 wks.	12 wks.	9 wks.
Viral antigens[e]						
Total	0	90.3	90.2	67.9	88.9	91.1
Preimmune	0	0	0	0	6.4	7.3
ICP 10	0	20.3	23.1	12.8	43.0	77.2
Preimmune	0	0	9.6	6.5	3.6	0

aLines established wiht pre-inactivated virus (HBU-1), or by exposure to nUV light at 4 (HT4A; HT4B), 6 (HT6A) or 8 (HT8A) hours p.i. PTP = post treatment passage.
b100 cells seeded/35mm dish and foci (> 40 cells) counted on day 10. Cloning efficiency (%) expressed as Number of colonies/Number cells seeded.
c10^4 cells seeded/35mm dish and colonies (> 20 cells) counted at 2 to 3 weeks. Cloning efficiency (%) expressed as Number of colonies x 100/10^4.
dNewborn hamsters were injected subcutaneously with 2 x 10^6 cells. Parentheses represent %.
ePercent complement fixed [5] by IgG from antisera to total viral proteins, ICP 10, or preimmune controls.

or to ICP 10 (Table 2). IgG from preimmune sera were non-reactive
(Table 4). The identity of the viral proteins responsible for the
reactivity of the cell extracts with antisera to total viral proteins
is unknown. However, besides ICP 10, which was common to all studied
transformants, 3 other proteins that co-migrate on SDS-acrylamide gel
electrophoresis with HSV-2 infected cell proteins ICP 7 (MW: 195,000),
ICP 22 (MW: 80,000), and ICP 35 (MW: 41,500) were observed in extracts
of HBU-1, HT4A, HT4B, and HT8A cells. Furthermore, late passage HT4A
and HT8A cells were positive for virus-specific cytoplasmic mRNA as
determined by in situ hybridization with a viral DNA probe free of
host cell DNA and viral RNA. Negative controls consisting of cells
transformed by B(a)P and normal SHE cells, were negative for viral
antigens/proteins and for viral RNA (Manak et al., in preparation).
Thus our studies confirm the conclusion [11-13] that HSV-2 transformants retain both a transformed phenotype and viral DNA sequences [20]
and argue against the "hit and run" hypothesis.

Given that: (i) the same pattern of BUdR substituted viral DNA
fragmentation occurs at all times post infection, and (ii) transformants (including those established with pre-inactivated virus) are positive at least for ICP 10, the $\geq$ 10 fold higher frequency of transformation observed between 4-8 hours p.i. (Table 3) appears to be due to
the expression of viral functions that are distinct from those (viz.
ICP 10) maintained in the transformed cells. These functions (hence-
forth designated "enhancer") are not a pre-requisite for transformation
since pre-inactivated virus or virus inactivated at 0 or 2 hours p.i.
retained its transforming potential. However, they increase the frequency of the transforming event(s) possibly by facilitating the integration of the "maintained" genes in the host cell DNA. Although the
identity of the "helper" functions is still unknown the observation
that the frequency of transformation did not increase in cells irradiated beyond 4 hours p.i. (Table 3) suggests that their synthesis had
already reached maximal levels by that time. Viral functions known
to be expressed by 4 hours p.i. include: (i) the induction of chromosomal lesions [21], (ii) inhibition of -amanitin sensitive RNA polymerase [22], (iii) increased thymidine metabolism such as transport

and phosyphorylation [23], and (iv) the stimulation of cell DNA synthesis [23].

Transforming HSV DNA sequences. Several recent reports have attempted
to localize the viral genes responsible for transformation. Camacho
and Spear [15], reported that viral DNA sequences contained in the
Xba I F fragment of HSV-1 DNA (map coordinates 20-45) are sufficient
to cause morphologic (but not tumorigenic) transformation of hamster
embryo cells as assayed by the ability of the transformed cells to
grow in low serum. The cells were originally positive for viral glycoproteins, however, were later found to be free of viral DNA sequences
[16]. Cells transfected with other HSV-1 DNA fragments also acquired
the ability to grow in low serum, but at a significantly lower frequency [15]. Reyes et al., [6] reported that transfection with a HSV-1
DNA fragment spanning map units 31-41 resulted in morphologic transformation of mouse cells as defined by focus formation. However the
focus inducing function of HSV-2 DNA was localized in the Bgl II N
fragment spanning map coordinates 58-63. Here again the cells were
not tumorigenic. On the other hand, HSV-2 DNA sequences capable of
inducing the neoplastic transformation of hamster embryo fibroblasts
were localized in the Bgl II/Hpa I CD fragment spanning map coordinates
43-58. Cells transformed by this fragment expressed viral antigens
(including ICP 10) for at least 60 passages [24].

Another approach [25] towards localization of the viral transforming sequences has been the identification of those viral DNA sequences
common to: (i) a cell line transformed by UV-inactivated HSV-2, (ii)
its clones and sub-clones, and (iii) two lines established from tumors
induced by one of these sub-clones. To this end, restriction endonuclease fragments of HSV-2 DNA spanning almost the entire genome were
isolated, made highly radioactive in vitro and a small amount was hybridized with large quantities of unlabeled DNA isolated from the
transformed and the tumor cells. Whereas the original transformed
line retained an extensive set of viral DNA sequences, a greatly decreased quantity was observed in sub-clones and particularly in the
tumor lines. Significantly, the only two blocks of viral DNA sequences

common to all the cells, including the two tumor lines, were those
homologous to the Ggl II G fragment (map units 21-33) and to the Xba
I D fragment. However, since sequences homologous to fragments that
overlap the right hand end of the Xba I D fragment (spanning map units
58-72) were not present in some of the lines, we conclude that only
those sequences spanning positions 45-58, overlapping virtually the
entire Bgl II/Hpa I CD fragment of Jariwalla et al., [24], were common
to all the lines.

From these results it is apparent that the location of the transforming HSV gene(s) remains unclear. Possibly the function assayed
by Camacho and Spear [15] and Reyes et al., [6] in their focus forma-
tion/low serum assay is a cell proliferation inducing function that
allows cells to grow in low serum but is unrelated to the putative
transforming gene. Indeed, we find that the frequency of transformation as assayed by the focus formation/low serum assay is significantly
($\geq$ 10 fold) higher than that observed in the continuous passage assay
(Table 3). However, since less than 10% of the isolated foci were
able to grow into stable lines, the relationship between this phenomenon and neoplastic potential remains to be established. Alternatively,
the function contained in the HSV-1 Xba I F fragment of Camacho and
Spear [15] and the HSV-2 Bgl II N fragment of Reys and co-workers [6],
may be only one of several functions required for stable HSV mediated
neoplastic transformation. Thus, one could visualize a stabilizer/
helper relationship between a putative transformation gene (VTR) and
"enhancer" gene (VH) located at another site on the genome (Figure 4),
that increases and/or stabilizes its transforming potential. That
such "helper" gene(s) do in fact exist in the HSV system is suggested
by our finding (Table 3) that the frequency of transformation is greatly increased by the expression of "early" viral gene(s) apparently
distinct from those maintained in the transformed cells. Similar conclusions were independently reached with other virus systems [26] and
in the HSV-induced biochemical transformation model [27].

Biochemical Transformation. Another type of HSV-mediated cell conversion involves the transfer of the HSV encoded tk gene to mouse cells

previously lacking this enzyme. This kind of biochemical conversion
was first demonstrated by Munyon et al., [14], who showed that following infection with UV-irradiated HSV, a small proportion of tk negative
(tk⁻) mouse cells survived selection in HAT containing medium because
they acquired and expressed the viral tk gene. The latter has been
mapped between coordinates 27 and 35 [28]. This finding is consistent
with those of Leiden et al., [29] who reported that although HSV-tk$^+$
transformants contain variable amounts of non-tk genes, the only DNA
sequences common to all transformants studied, were those located between map coordinated 28 and 32. Analyses of several HSV-tk$^+$ cell
lines differing in the stability of their tk phenotype have indicated
that most likely both the expression of the HSV tk gene (in selective
medium) and the stability of this expression during cell propagation
in non-selective medium are under cellular rather than viral control.
Indeed, an identical set of viral DNA sequences located between map
coordinates 23 and 31 were found in a HSV-1 tk$^+$ transformed cell line,
a tk⁻ revertant and a tk$^+$ re-revertant indicating that reversion and
re-reversion of the HSV-tk$^+$ phenotype does not appear to involve
changes in viral DNA content [16]. Although the exact mechanism where-
by reversion of the tk$^+$ phenotype occurs without any changes in the
complexity of cell associated viral DNA is unknown, it should be pointed out that the reversion mechanism may vary as a function of the selection method. Thus Kraiselburd et al., [30] have shown that a tk⁻
revertant of a HSV tk$^+$ line selected by growth in BUdR containing
medium, lost all detectable HSV DNA sequences.

Progression/Selection. As previously reported for cells transformed
by B(a)P or by perturbation to cellular DNA [7-9], SHE cells transformed with HSV-2 inactivated by the BUdR and nUV ligh procedure demonstrated morphologic alterations and growth in low serum at post-treatment passage (ptp)4-8 (Figure 1), entered crisis at ptp 8-10, and re-
covered at ptp 12-24. This interval was characterized by a doubling
time reduced to 12-16 hours, as compared to the 20-24 hrs. for SHE
cells. Anchorage independence was first detected at ptp 24-37 and
increased with cell passage (Figure 2A). Its appearance was virtually

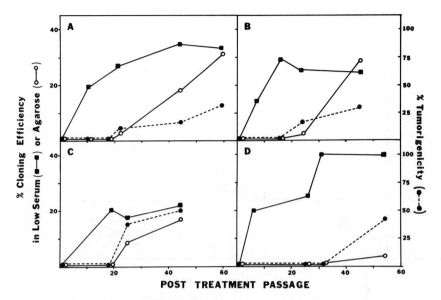

Figure 1. Temporal acquisition of altered growth characteristics in HSV-2 induced transformants HBU-5 (A), HT4C (B), HT4A (C), and HBU-3 (D), examined at various ptp. ■———■ cloning efficiency in low serum; o----o cloning efficiency in 0.3% agarose; ●———● tumor incidence (%).

concommittant (ptp 24-54) with the acquisition of tumorigenic potential for newborn hamsters (Figure 1).

This temporal acquisition of the transformed phenotype appears to be due to a progressive passage of the cells through qualitatively different stages, since clones isolated at early (ptp 8) or intermediate (ptp 25) passage did not express anchorage independence until they independently reached ptp 35-55 (Figure 2B). However, it should be pointed out that not all cells within a population reach the same qualitative stage at the same time. Thus, two clones isolated at passage (ptp 35), when the parental line already expressed a 5% cloning efficiency in 0.3% agarose, differed in their ability to grow in semi-solid medium. One of them (HBU-1 Ag) demonstrated a 20% cloning efficiency within 3 independent passages whereas the other (HBU-1 AA) reached similar cloning efficiency only at ptp 55 (Figure 2B).

Unlike growth in low serum, anchorage independence correlates well with tumorigenicity both in the hamster (Figure 1) and the rat [12] systems. Significantly, although expression of ICP 10 preceded anchorage independence by 13-17 passages, we found that it is strongly

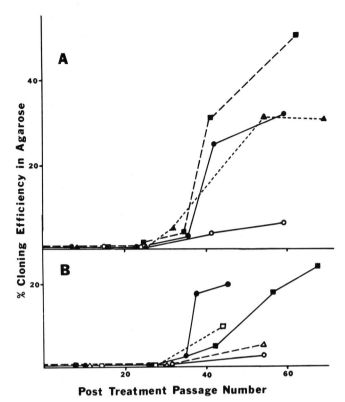

Figure 2. Acquisition of anchorage independence (% cloning efficienty in 0.3% agarose) by: (A) HSV-2 transformed lines HT-8 ■ ; HBU-1 ● ; HT-6 ▲ ; HBU-4 ○ , and (B) clones derived from HBU at ptp 19 (○ HBU-1EA) and at ptp 35 (● HBU-1Ag; ■ HBU-1AA) and clones derived from HT4B at ptp 15: (□ HT-4B Cl; △ HT-4B Cl ¹).

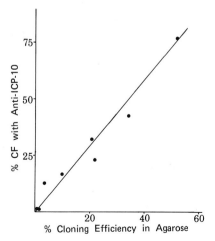

Figure 3. Relation between cloning efficiency in 0.3% agarose at late (> 40) ptp and the expression (% CF) of viral protein ICP 10.

correlated with the acquisition of anchorage independence (99% confidence level, $p \leq 0.01$ according to Kendall's coefficient of rank correlation). This analysis (Figure 3) includes two morphologically altered lines capable of growing in low serum but not in 0.3% agarose, that are both ICP 10 negative and non-tumorigenic. A similar correlation was not observed with respect to total viral antigens (Table 4), suggesting that although transformants express viral proteins other than ICP 10, these are not related to anchorage independence. An interesting exception to the apparent correlation of tumorigenicity and anchorage independence is a line of HSV-2 transformed rat cells that displays anchorage independence but is not-tumorigenic. This line becomes tumorigenic upon exposure to the tumor promoting agent 12-0-tetradecanoyl-phorbol-13-acetate (TPA), concomittant with the expression of a protein, not hitherto expressed, that is identical in molecular weight to ICP 10 (Kucera, personal communication).

Unlike the progression hypothesis that interprets the in vitro acquisition of a neoplastic potential as resulting from a progressive passage of the cells through qualitatively different stages, the selection hypothesis argues that a small number of fully transformed cells is already present in a cell population at an early ptp, however its detection is masked by a larger number of normal cells. In support of this interpretation, Kucera [12] showed that foci of HSV-2 transformed rat cells at early passage produce small numbers of colonies in soft agar. Lines established from these soft agar colonies were then shown to be tumorigenic, thus obviating the requirement for long (up to 2 years) in vivo latent periods described for low passage rat transformants [31]. This prolonged in vivo latent period was also significantly reduced by exposure of the transformed rat cells to the tumor promoting agent TPA (Kucera, L., personal communication).

Mechanism of Transformation: A Unified Hypothesis

Presently available data on regulatory aspects of cell division, and the information on virus and chemical induced transformation, can be used to develop the general outline of a unified hypothesis of the mechanism of transformation. The basic assumptions are as follows:

POSITIVE CONTROL

NORMAL

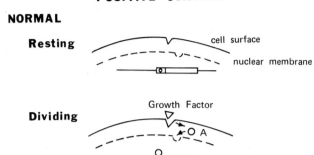

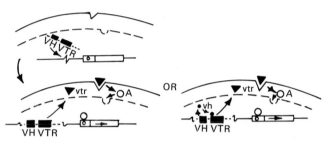

Figure 4. Schematic representation of the hypothetical mechanism of virus induced transformation, according to the positive control of DNA synthesis cell division. A regulatory host-encoded cytoplasmic factor (A), posited as the activator of DNA synthesis/cell division, is induced by the interaction of growth factors with the cell surface. It acts directly on the operator (O) of the gene regulating DNA synthesis or by interaction with the nuclear membrane. Transformation is visualized as resulting from an imbalance in growth regulation. It is postulated that a virus gene (VTR) codes for a transforming protein (vtr) that: (i) mimicks the action of the growth factors thus inducing activator (A) molecules, or (ii) mimicks the action of the activator itself (not shown). Another viral gene (VH) that is not absolutely necessary for transformation and may or may not be retained in transformed cells, significantly enhances transformation frequency by producing a "helper" protein (vh). This protein acts by stabilizing the VTR gene in the host cells (integration) or by turning on the "maintained" VTR gene.

(i) All carcinogens induce neoplastic transformation via a similar molecular pathway independent of their original interaction with the cell, (ii) DNA synthesis/cell division is a pivotal event in the progression of a cell towards a state of neoplastic transformation, (iii) DNA synthesis/cell division is regulated by cell surface triggers, such as those functionally identified by altered growth characteristics and (iv) a finite number of regulatory molecules, most probably cell encoded, are required in order to control DNA synthesis/cell division, and they are synthesized in a limited number.

Regulatory Aspects of Cell Division. The cell cycle can be divided into 4 classical phases: G1, S (DNA synthesis period), G2, and M (mitosis). In addition, cells can exist in a non-growing quiescent state (GO) in which they do not divide [32]. The point in the cell cycle at which cells make a committment to divide or to enter (GO) is called the restriction point and occurs near the middle of the G1 phase. Once the restriction point is passed, the cell is irreversibly committed to undergo a series of events including the initiation of DNA synthesis, membrane alterations, and ultimately cell division. Regulation of the restriction point in normal cells is subject to environmental constraints such as imposed by the presence in the medium, of serum, hormones or certain nutrients, or by contact with substrate or with other cells.

Two hypotheses have been advanced for the regulation of cell division. The first is by means of an activator of DNA synthesis (A) and will be termed positive control (Figure 4). The second is by means of a repressor (R) of cell division and will be termed negative control (Figure 5). Transformation can be viewed as a defect in the regulation of the restriction point such that cells are continuously stimulated to divide (positive control) or are unable to enter the GO phase (negative control) (Figures 4, 5).

In the normal cells, the rate of synthesis of the postulated activator of DNA synthesis (A) may be under the control of various extracellular growth factors such as serum, hormones, epidermal growth factor (EGF), multiplication stimulating activity (MSA), and others [33].

NEGATIVE CONTROL

NORMAL

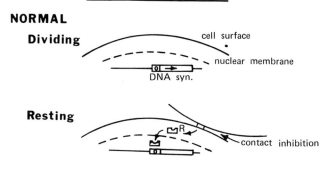

TRANSFORMED

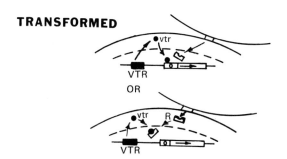

Figure 5. Schematic representation of the hypothetical mechanism of virus-induced transformation according to the negative control of cell division. According to this interpretation, a repressor (R) of DNA synthesis, subject to modulation by external factors (viz. contact inhibition), acts by binding the DNA (0) thus preventing its replication (resting cells). Virus transformed cells produce a transforming protein (vtr) that is encoded by the viral gene (VTR) and blocks the repressor (R) by binding it or its DNA attachment site. As discussed in Figure 4, VTR may interact with another viral gene (VH) (not shown).

Indeed, such factors bind to specific plasma membrane receptors and stimulate DNA synthesis in quiescent cells [34,35]. The response of cells to these external stimuli appears to be mediated by a cytoplasmic activator of DNA synthesis. Such a cytoplasmic mediator has been shown to be produced in hormone-stimulated cells, and to be capable of inducing DNA synthesis in vitro in isolated nuclei [35,36]. Studies

of hybrids of cells in early G1 with those in late G1 suggest that
this activator of DNA synthesis accumulates throughout the G1 phase,
and when a critical level of this activator is reached, the cells are
committed to DNA synthesis and therefore cell division [37]. In addition, it has been shown that both dividing and transformed cells secrete plasminogen activator (PA) which can stimulate resting cells
(in GO) to divide. This stimulation may be due to the potentiation
of the action of growth factors, or to the proteolytic alteration of
cell membrane-associated proteins. For example, secreted, membrane-
associated protein LETS, is lost during rapid growth periods but re-
appears concomittant with a decrease of PA secretion, in density inhibited cells [38].

     Although not as strong, evidence in support of the negative hy-
pothesis (Figure 5) has also accumulated. Thus, density inhibited
cells were shown to secrete membrane constituents, such as a glycoprotein [39] or mucosaccharide [40], that restore transformed cells
(melanocytes and hepatocytes) to density inhibition of growth. This
observation suggests that transformed cells are incapable of secreting
a repressor of cell division, although they can still respond to such
an inhibitor when added exogenuously. In another study, it was found
that a surface membrane fraction from normal murine (3T3) cells inhibits the rate of DNA synthesis in normal, but not in SV40 transformed
3T3 cells [41]. Similar membrane preparations from transformed cells
had a significantly less inhibitory effect on DNA synthesis in normal
cells suggesting that transformed cells failed both to produce and
to respond to an inhibitor of DNA synthesis.

     The surface membrane appears to play a major role in the regula-
tion of cell division, both in terms of its response to exogenous
stimulating/inhibitory factors, and the production of intracellular
activators/repressors of DNA synthesis. Thus numerous alterations
in cell surface are observed during periods of rapid cell division
in normal cells including lectin-induced agglutinability and expression
of receptor sites [42], membrane lipid fluidity [43], transport processes, electrical properties, and activities of membrane bound enzyme
[44]. Since all these activities are interrelated, loss or alteration

of one or a few membrane proteins could have pleiotropic effects on
the behavior of many surface proteins influencing their interaction
with each other and with the interior of the cell.

Transformation. In the previous sections, we have discussed presently
available information on cell transformation by HSV-2 and DNA perturbations. Are these conditions unique or can the information be gen-
eralized? The evidence supports generalization and is schematically
diagrammed in Figures 4-6. Thus, transformation of mammalian cells
by viruses generally requires the maintenance and expression of specific viral transforming gene(s) (designated VTR in Figure 4), and
chemical-induced transformation is more complex than a single mutational event (Figure 6). For example, the RNA tumor viruses contain a
transformation-specific gene (sarc) [45] that codes for a protein responsible for generation of the transformed phenotype [46]. The sarc
gene product, a stimulator of DNA synthesis [47], localizes on the
membranes of transformed cells and mimicks the effect of growth factors
[48]. Continued expression of this transforming protein is required
for maintenance of transformed and tumorigenic characteristics, as
evidenced by the observation [49] that cells transformed by temperature-
sensitive (ts) mutants of the sarc gene, when shifted to non-permissive
temperatures revert to normal growth controls and tumor regression.
The generation of a transformed phenotype by the DNA tumor viruses
involves a number of viral proteins with interlocking regulatory constraints, and their interaction with a host protein. Thus, cells transformed by SV40 express 2 virus-specific tumor antigens, T (94,000
daltons) predominantly nuclear, and t (20,000 daltons) predominantly
cytoplasmic, as well as a cell encoded tumor antigen (NVT, 50-56,000
daltons) all of which are precipitated by sera from tumor-bearing animals [50]. In SV40 transformed cells (but not in productively infected
cells) a stable association is observed between T and NVT [51] believed
to be responsible for the induction of cell DNA synthesis in arrested
cells [52]. Synthesis of T antigen in turn appears to be regulated
by another viral gene product normally expressed early in infection.

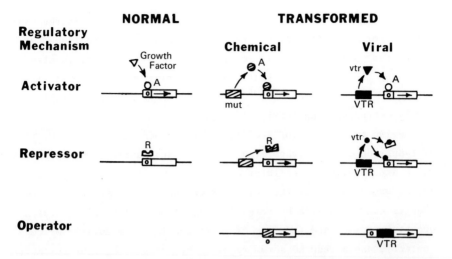

Figure 6. Comparative representation of transformation induced by virus or chemical carcinogens. Uncontrolled production of the activator (A) of DNA synthesis (positive control) results from a mutation (▨) in the cellular gene coding for A (chemical) or from the integration and continuous expression of the VTR (Figure 4) gene (viral). According to the negative control theory, alteration of the repressor (R) of DNA synthesis by mutation (chemical) in the repressor gene (▨) or by the production (viral) of vtr (Figure 5) result in uncontrolled cell DNA synthesis/division. Under certain conditions, transformation may also result from the alteration of the operator region of the gene regulating DNA synthesis (0) by mutation (▨) or by VTR insertion such that DNA synthesis is no longer subject to regulation by R or A.

In support of this conclusion are data generated with a ts mutant of the SV40 transformation gene. One type of transformant induced by this mutant, designated type N, loses T-antigen expression and reverts back to normal growth regulation when shifted to the non-permissive temperature, although it retains viral DNA sequences coding for T-antigen. The second type of transformant generated with the ts mutant, designated type A, retains both the expression of T-antigen and its transformed phenotype at both the permissive and non-permissive temperatures [53]. The data indicate that although both transformant types maintain the DNA sequences coding for T-antigen, the requirement for the virus regulatory protein that normally modulates the expression of T-antigen is somehow bypassed in type A cells. That viral proteins other than T-antigen may play an important role in the expression and/or stabilization of transformation by SV40 or polyoma, although they are not strictly required for transformation, is also supported by the observation that viable deletion mutants mapping in the 0.54-0.59 region of the SV40 [26] or polyoma [54] genomes display severely depressed transforming frequencies.

Using ts mutants for t-antigen, it has been shown that the role of t-antigen in SV40 transformation is to de-stabilize the actin cables which are involved in cellular adhesion, mobility, morphology, and in the organization of the cell surface [63]. Significantly, these changes correlate with PA release (transformed cells secrete large quantities of PA and the rate of secretion is not modulated by cell contact), and a reduced serum requirement for growth, thus resembling those changes observed in normal cells exposed to EGF. It may be concluded that transformation by SV40 probably involves the coordinate effect of: (i) t antigen which disrupts the normal organization of cellular structure and control thus permitting a stable integration of the transforming gene(s), and (ii) T-antigen (interacting with NVT) a regulator of DNA synthesis that ultimately accounts for the tumorigenic characteristics of the cells.

Transformation by other DNA tumor viruses likewise involves more than one viral function. Cells transformed by adenovirus express at least two tumor antigens; a small cell surface polypeptide of 16,000 daltons [55], and a 60,000 dalton protein that binds native, but not denatured DNA [56]. These proteins are coded by a subset of early viral genes mapping at the left-most 7.2% of the viral genome [64] that presumably act to maintain a transformed phenotype. As with SV40, the synthesis of the transforming proteins of adenovirus, is regulated by early viral proteins. Viral polypeptides made early after infection with adenovirus regulate synthesis of all the early RNA's including the one (22 S RNA) coding for the transforming proteins [57]. Increased accumulation of 22S RNA requires the presence of a protein specific for the stimulation of 22S RNA and the absence of the unstable polypeptide which regulates negatively all the early RNA's.

Transforming functions of polyoma and adenovirus have been shown to reside in two complementation groups. One of these (Adeno 5 hr II [58], and polyoma hrt [59]) is not required for viral DNA synthesis in certain cells, but is necessary for initiation of transformation. The other complementation group (adeno 5 hr I, and polyoma tsA) is required for viral DNA synthesis and possibly for the maintenance of a transformed phenotype. Transformation by viruses having a defect in this second complementation group is abortive. Thus, these defective viruses induce morphologically altered colonies but most of these regress and fail to establish stable lines. The few lines that can be passed for extended periods of time and that exhibit some of the transformed characteristics, are consistently non-tumorigenic.

The data discussed in an earlier section support the conclusion that HSV-2 induced neoplastic transformation, though not as well studied as yet, also requires the contribution of at least two types of functions that we have respectively designated "enhancer" and "maintenance". Furthermore, in the biochemical transformation system it has recently been shown, using ts mutants of HSV-1, that the frequency of stable tk transformation is greatly enhanced by the expression of another viral gene product(s) that maps outside the tk region. This gene (spanning map coordinates 30-60) is required for viral DNA synthesis and is expressed early in the course of viral infection. Although it is not absolutely required for tk transformation, its expression can greatly enhance the frequency of the tk transformation [27].

Since, as discussed in a previous section, transformation induced by chemical carcinogens or by direct perturbation to cell DNA appears to be more complex than a single mutational event, our hypothesis postulates that it involves the induction following an original mutation, of an interlocking cascading set of events (Figure 6). This set of events ultimately results in the irreversible committment of the cell to DNA synthesis/division by processes similar to those summarized in Figures 4, 5. It should be pointed out that our hypothesis does not exclude the possibility that transformation could occur as the result of a single mutational event or by the simple incorporation

of viral gene(s) in absence of expression, provided that these occur
in the operator for cell division (Figure 6).

How does our hypothesis contend with the observation that tumorigenicity is acquired as a progressive passage through qualitatively
different stages? The expression of a transformed phenotype such as
PA secretion (from membrane), reduced serum requirement (altered membrane receptors for growth factors), loss of contact inhibition (membrane mediated cell to cell communication), anchorage independent
growth (membrane attachment to surface), and tumorigenicity (alteration of cell surface so as to become unresponsive to growth controls,
and insensitive to the immune system) can be considered different
stages in the alteration of cell membranes. Given that all these membrane effects are inter-related, it may be postulated (Figure 7), that
the progressive acquisition of morphologic alterations, growth in low
serum, anchorage independence and tumorigenicity, represents the progressive loss of response to R (negative control hypothesis of cell
division) or the progressive accumulation of A (positive control of
cell division) (Figures 4, 5). According to this interpretation, the
initial transforming event would produce an imbalance in the rate of
production of A or R per cell cycle, but time and subsequent cell divisions would be required before the full effect of this imbalance
can be observed (Figure 7). Assuming that: (i) a finite number of
regulatory molecules (A or R) are essential in order to regulate cell
DNA synthesis, and (ii) those functions associated with neoplastic
transformation, (such as morphologic alteration, growth in low serum,
and anchorage independence), are controlled by cellular genes that
are contiguously regulated, it follows that quantitative defects in
regulatory molecules would de-regulate the expression of these genes
in a cascading, interlocking order. Alternatively, it may be argued
that at consecutive stages in its life cycle, the cell is faced with
a multiple choice such as, for example, growth in low serum vs. increased volume. The cumulative effect of these choices will determine
the cell's ultimate fate in immortality or senescence.

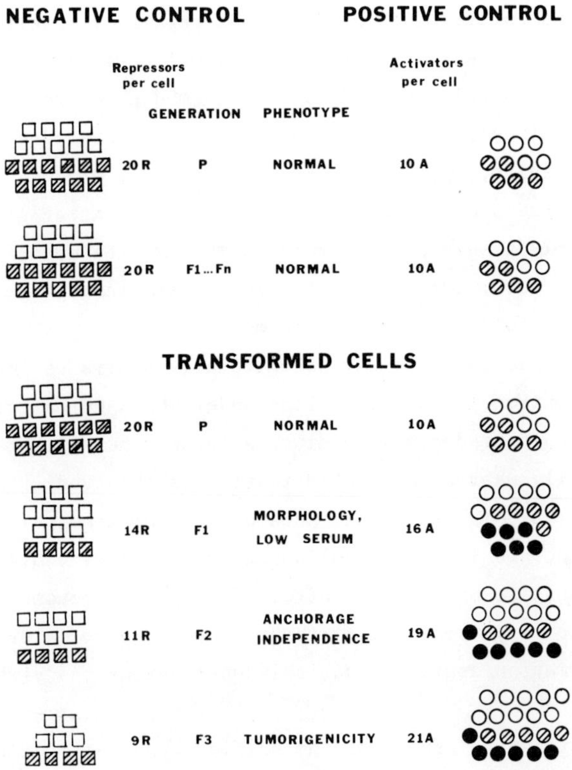

Figure 7. Schematic representation of the "progression" hypothesis for the acquisition of a transformed phenotype. It is postulated that a finite number of regulatory molecules (20 R or 10 A) are required to control DNA synthesis/cell division. With each generation (F_1-F_n), half of the regulator molecules are inherited by each daughter cell (□ ○ parental), while the others are newly synthesized (▨ ◙). In transformed cells, the synthesis and/or activity of the regulator molecules (R/A) are altered. A reduced number/activity of R molecules or an increased number/activity of A molecules (5 newly made ○ + 6 virus induced ●) are made at each cell division. Due to the presence of parental R/A at early ptp (F_1) the end-point of transformation (tumorigenicity) is not expressed. However, contiguously controlled early changes, such as morphologic alteration and reduced serum requirements are observed. An intermediate ptp (F_2) as the amount of parental R is diluted out or the amount of A increases, the cellular changes become more pronounced (anchorage independence). In the final stages of transformation (here designated F_3) the amount of R/A has stabilized at levels leading to a permanent loss in the regulation of cell division and to tumorigenicity.

Numerous observations suggest that regulatory controls of cell division that are unrelated to the original carcinogen/virus, are involved in the establishment of a transformed phenotype. Thus rapidly growing normal cells present in a population containing only a few transformed cells, appear to have an inhibitory effect of the expression of the transformed characteristics of the latter group, particularly at early stages after carcinogen/virus treatment. Cells maintained in 5% serum for the first 2 weeks after carcinogen treatment, exhibit a 2-6 fold greater transformation frequency than those maintained in 10% serum while 20% serum totally abolishes the expression of transformation [60]. Conditions under which normal cells rapidly die off in calcium-depleted medium, allow morphologic transformation by Ad 5 hr II, whereas no transformation is observed if normal cells are allowed to persist for extended periods of time [61]. If cells are maintained in low serum following treatment with SV40 tsA, transformation that is under the control of the viral genome ensues, but if cells are permitted to proliferate in 10% serum, a different type of transformation appears that is independent of the viral genome [62].

The attractive aspect of the unified hypothesis of transformation presented in this report, is that it is amenable to experimental verification. Much is already known about the role of the relatively small viruses (SV40, adenovirus, sarcoma viruses) in the regulation and control of cellular events resulting in a transforming phenotype. However, with respect to large complex viruses that, like HSV-2, have been associated with human carcinogenesis, significant questions (detailed in previous sections) remain unanswered. The evidence that direct DNA perturbation will lead to neoplastic transformation, underscores the role of the cell in its ultimate fate - immortality or senescence. However, so far, there is no evidence that this specific perturbation results, as postulated by our hypothesis, in a cascading set of perturbations to other target molecules. As technology develops, the verification of the questions raised and the predictions made by the unified hypothesis of transformation should provide new insights into mechanistic aspects that have direct bearing on human

disease. The implications that such interpretations have on differ-
entiation/control, cancer, and ultimately the molecular biology of
the mammalian genetic apparatus, constitute one of the major, present
challenges to the intellectual activities of man.

ACKNOWLEDGMENTS

Studies done in our laboratory were supported by Program Project Grant
CA 16043 from the National Cancer Institute. We thank Mrs. J. Roberson
for help with the manuscript.

REFERENCES

1. Koss, L. G., Concept of genesis and development of carcinoma of
    the cervis, *Obst. Gynec. Survey, 24*:850-860 (1969).

2. Rawls, W. E., and Adam, E., Hepres simplex viruses and human
    malignancies. In: Origin of Human Cancer - Mechanisms of Car-
    cinogenesis. Hiatt, H. H., Watson, J. D., and Winston, J. A.,
    eds. Cold Spring Harbor Conference on Cell Proliferation, Vol.
    4, pp. 1133-1155, 1977.

3. Aurelian, L., Jariwalla, R. J., Kessler, I. I., and Ts'o, P. O. P.,
    Herpes simplex virus type 2 and cervical cancer: cells trans-
    formed by a viral DNA fragment express the cervical tumor-asso-
    ciated antigen AG-4. In: Viruses in Naturally Occurring Cancers.
    Essex, M., Todaro, G., and ZurHausen, H., eds. Cold Spring Harbor
    Conferences on Cell Proliferation, Vol. 7, 1980, in press.

4. McDougall, J. K., Fenoglio, C. M., and Galloway, D. A., Detection
    of Herpes simplex virus RNA in latently infected ganglion cells
    and in cervical neoplasia. In: Viruses in Naturally Occurring
    Cancers. Essex, M., Todaro, G., and ZurHausen, H., eds. Cold
    Spring Harbor Conferences on Cell Proliferation, Vol. 7, 1980,
    in press.

5. Aurelian, L., Strnad, B. C., and Smith, M. F., Immunodiagnostic
    potential of virus-coded tumor-associated antigen (AG-4) in
    cervical cancer, *Cancer, 39*:1834-1849 (1977).

6. Reyes, G. R., LaFemina, R., Hayward, S. D., and Hayward, G. S.,
    Transforming fragments of HSV DNA, *Cold Spring Harbor Symp.
    Quant. Biol., 44*, in press.

7. Ts'o, P. O. P., Neoplastic transformation, somatic mutation and differentiation. Carcinogenesis: Fundamental Mechanisms and Environmental Effects. In: Proc. 13th Jerusalem Symposia on Quantum Chemistry and Biochemistry. Reidel, D., ed. Dordercht, Holland, in press.

8. Barret, J. C., Crawford, B., Nixter, L., Schechtman, L., Ts'o, P. and Pollack, R., Correlation of in vitro growth properties and tumorigenicity of Syrian hamster cell lines, *Cancer Res., 39:*1504-1510 (1979).

9. Barrett, J. C. and Ts'o, P. O. P., Relationship between somatic mutation and neoplastic transformation, *Proc. Nat. Acad. Sci., 75:*3297-3301 (1978).

10. Tsutsui, T., Barrett, J. C., and Ts'o, P. O. P., Morphological transformation DNA damage and chromosal aberration induced by a direct DNA perturbation of synchronized Syrian hamster embryo cells, *Cancer Res., 39:*2356-2365 (1979).

11. Duff, R., and Rapp, F., Properties of hamster embryo fibroblasts transformed in vitro after exposure to ultraviolet irradiated herpes simplex virus type 2, *J. Virol., 8:*469-477 (1971).

12. Kucera, L. A., Gusdon, J. P., Edwards, I., and Herbst, G., Oncogenic transformation of rat embryo fibroblasts with photoinactivated herpes simplex virus: rapid in vitro cloning of transformed cells, *J. Gen. Virol., 35:*473-485 (1977).

13. Darai, F., and Munk, K., Human embryonic lung cells abortively infected with herpes virus hominis type 2 show some properties of cell transformation, *Nature New Biol., 241:*268-269 (1973).

14. Munyon, W., Kraiselburd, E., Davis, D., and Mann, J., Transfer of thymidine kinase to thymidine kinaseless L cells by infection with UV-irradiated herpes simplex virus, *J. Virol., 7:*813-820 (1971).

15. Camacho, A., and Spear, P. G., Transformation of hamster embryo fibroblasts by a specific fragment of the herpes simplex virus genome, *Cell, 15:*993-1002 (1978).

16. Leiden, J. and Frenkel, N., Mapping of the herpes simplex virus sequences in transformed cells. In: Herpes virus DNA: Recent Studies of the Viral Genome. Y. Becker et al., ed., in press.

17. Hampar, B., and Boyd, A., Interaction of oncornaviruses and herpes viruses: a hypothesis proposing a co-carcinogenic role for herpes viruses in transformation, A Review. In: Oncogenesis and Herpes viruses III, Part 2, Cell Virus Interactions, Host Response to Herpes virus Infection and Associated Tumors, Rold of Co-Factors. deThe, G., Henle, W., and Rapp, F., eds. LARC Publications, Lyon France, 1978.

18. Dulbecco, R., Topoinhibition and serum requirement of transformed and untransformed cells, *Nature, 227*:802-806 (1970).

19. Jariwalla, R., Aurelian, L., and Ts'o, P. O. P., Neoplastic transformation of cultured syrian hamster embryo cells by DNA of herpes simplex virus type 2, *J. Virol., 30*:404-409 (1979).

20. Frenkel, N., Locker, H., Cox, B., Roizman, B., and Rapp, F., Herpes simplex virus DNA in transformed cells: sequency complexity in five hamster cell lines and one derived hamster tumor, *J. Virol., 18*:885-893 (1976).

21. Oneil, F., and Rapp, R., Early events required for induction of chromosome abnormalities in human cells by HSV, *Virol., 44*:544-553 (1971).

22. Preston, C., and Newton, A., The effects of HSV-1 on cellular DNA-dependent RNA polymerase activities, *J. Gen. Virol., 33*:471-482 (1976).

23. Kucera, L., and Edwards, I., HSV type 2 functions expressed during stimulation of human cell DNA, *J. Virol., 29*:83-90 (1979).

24. Jariwalla, R. J., Aurelian, L., and Ts'o, P. O. P., Tumorigenic transformation induced by a specific fragment of herpes simplex virus type 2 DNA, *Proc. Nat. Acad. Sci., U.S.A., 77*:2279-2238 (1980).

25. Galloway, D. A., Copple, C. D., McDougall, J. K., Analysis of viral DNA sequences in hamster cells transformed by herpes simplex virus type 2, *Proc. Nat. Acad. Sci., U.S.A., 77*:880-884 (1980).

26. Feunteum, Kress, M., Gardes, M., and Monier, R., Viable deletion mutants in the Simian virus 40 early region, *Proc. Nat. Acad. Sci., U.S.A., 75*:4455-4459 (1978).

27. Rapp, F., Turner, N., and Schaffer, P., Biochemical transformation by temperature-sensitive mutants of herpes simplex virus type 1, *J. Virol., 34*:704-710 (1980).

28. Wigler, M., Silverstein, S., Lee, Sih-Syng, Pellicer, A., Cheng, Yung-chi, and Axel, R., Transfer of purified herpes virus thymidine kinase gene to cultured mouse cells, *Cell, 11*:223-232 (1977).

29. Leiden, J. M., Frenkel, N., and Rapp, F., Identification of the herpes simplex virus DNA sequences present in six herpes simplex virus thymidine kinase transformed mouse cell lines, *J. Virol., 33*:272-285 (1980).

30. Kraiselburd, E., Gage, L. P., Weissbach, A., Presence of a herpes simplex virus DNA fragment in an L cell clone obtained after infection with irradiated herpes simplex virus type 1, *J. Mol. Biol., 97*:533-542 (1975).

31. McNab, J., Tumor production by HSV-2 transformed lines in rats and the varying response to immunosuppression, *J. Gen. Virol.*, *22*:1317-1334 (1979).

32. Pardee, A., A restriction point for control of normal animal cell proliferation, *Proc. Nat. Acad. Sci.*, *U.S.A.*, *71*:1286-1290 (1974).

33. Gospodarowicz, D., and Moran, J., Growth factors in Mammalian cell culture, *Ann. Rev. Biochem.*, *45*:531-558 (1976).

34. Rechler, M., Podskalny, J., and Nissley, S., Interaction of multiplication stimulating activity with chick embryo fibroblasts demonstrates a growth receptor, *Nature*, *259*:134-136 (1976).

35. Das, M., Mitogenic hormone induced intracellular message: assay and partial characterization of an activator of DNA replication induced by epidermal growth factor, *Proc. Nat. Acad. Sci.*, *U.S.A.*, *77*:112-116 (1980).

36. Benblow, R., and Ford, C., Cytoplasmic control of nuclear DNA synthesis during early development of Xenopus Laevis: A cell-free assay, *Proc. Nat. Acad. Sci.*, *U.S.A.*, *72*:2437-2441 (1975).

37. Rao, R., Sunkara, P., and Wilson, B., Regulation of DNA synthesis: Age dependent cooperation among G1 cells upon fusion, *Proc. Nat. Acad. Sci.*, *U.S.A.*, *74*:2869-2873 (1977).

38. Chou, I., O'Donnell, S., Black, P., and Robin, R., Cell density-dependent secretion of plasminogen activator by 3T3 cells, *J. Cell. Physiol.*, *91*:31-37 (1977).

39. Lipkin, G., and Krecht, M., Contact inhibition of growth is restored to malignant melanocytes of man and mouse by a hamster protein, *Exp. Cell. Res.*, *102*:341-348 (1976).

40. Ohnishi, T., Ohshima, E., and Ohtusuka, M., Effect of liver cell coat acid mucopolysaccharide on the appearance of density-dependent inhibition in hepatoma cell growth, *Exp. Cell. Res.*, *93*:136-147 (1975).

41. Whittenberger, B., and Glaser, L., Inhibition of DNA synthesis in cultures of 3T3 cells by isolated surface membranes, *Proc. Nat. Acad. Sci.*, *U.S.A.*, *74*:2251-2255 (1977).

42. Nicolson, G., Transmembrane control of the receptors on normal and tumor cells. I. Cytoplasmic influence over cell surface components, *Biochem. Biophys. Acta.*, *457*:57-108 (1976).

43. deLaat, S., van der Saag, P., Elson, E., and Schlessinger, J., Lateral diffusion of membrane lipids and proteins during the cell cycle of neuroblastoma cells, *Proc. Nat. Acad. Sci.*, *U.S.A.*, *77*:1526-1528 (1980).

44. Schlessinger, J., Schechter, J., and Cuatracacas, Y., Quantitative determination of the lateral diffusion coefficients of the hormone-receptor complexes of insulin and epidermal growth factor on the plasma membrane of cultured fibroblasts, *Proc. Nat. Acad. Sci., U.S.A., 75*:5353-5357 (1978).

45. Duesberg, P., and Vogt, P., RNA species obtained from clonal lines of Avian sarcoma and from avian leukosis virus, *Virology, 54*:207-219 (1973).

46. Bernstein, A., MacCormich, R., and Martin, G., Transformation-defective mutants of Avian sarcoma viruses: the genetic relationship between conditional and nonconditional mutants, *Virology, 70*:206-209 (1976).

47. Todaro, G., DeLarco, J., and Cohen, S., Transformation by murine and feline sarcoma viruses specifically blocks binding of epidermal growth factor to cells, *Nature, 264*:26-28 (1976).

48. Willingham, M., Pastan, I., Shih, T., and Scolnick, E., Localization of the src gene product of the Harvey strain of MSV to plasma membrane of transformed cells by electron microscopic immunobhemistry, *Cell, 19*:1005-1014 (1980).

49. Klarund, J., and Forchhammer, J., Temperature-sensitive tumorigenicity of cells transformed by a mutant of Maloney sarcoma virus, *Proc. Nat. Acad. Sci., U.S.A., 77*:1501-1505 (1980).

50. Simmons, D., Martin, M., Mora, P., and Chang, C., Relationship among Tau antigens isolated from various lines of Simian virus 40-transformed cells, *J. Virol., 34*:650-657 (1980).

51. McCormick, F., and Harlow, E., Association of a murine 53,000 dalton phosphoprotein with Simian virus 40 large T antigen in transformed cells, *J. Virol., 34*:213-224 (1980).

52. Graessman, M., and Graessman, A., "Early" Simian-virus-40-specific RNA contains information for tumor antigen formation and chromatin replication, *Proc. Nat. Acad. Sci., U.S.A., 73*:366-370 (1976).

53. Gaudray, P., Rassoulzadeyan, M., and Cuzin, F., Expression of Simian virus 40 early genes in transformed rat cells is correlated with the maintenance of the transformed phenotype, *Proc. Nat. Acad. Sci., U.S.A., 75*:4987-4991 (1978).

54. Sleigh, M., Topp, W., Hanich, R., and Sambrook, J, Mutants of SV40 with an altered small t protein are reduced in there ability to transform cells, *Cell, 14*:79-88 (1978).

55. Vasconcelos-Costa, J., Solubilization and purification of surface antigen of cells transformed by adenovirus type 12, *Virol., 71*:122-133 (1976).

56. Biron, K., and Raska, K., Jr., Purification of adenovirus type
    12 tumor antigens from transformed hamster cells, *Virol.*, *76*:516-
    525 (1977).

57. Eggerding, F., and Raskas, H., Regulation of early RNA transcribed
    from the transforming segment of the adenovirus 2 genome, *Virol.*,
    91:312-320 (1978).

58. Graham, F., Harrison, T., and Williams, J., Defective transforming
    capacity of adenovirus type 5 host-range mutants, *Virol.*, *86*:10-
    21 (1978).

59. Eckhart, W., Complementation between temperature-sensitive (ts)
    and host range non-transforming (hr-t) mutants of polyoma virus,
    Virol., *77*:589-597 (1977).

60. Bertram, J., Effects of serum concentration on the expression
    of carcinogen-induced transformation in the C3H/10T 1/2 CL8 cell
    line, *Cancer Res.*, *37*:514-523 (1977).

61. Graham, F., Harrison, T., and Williams, J., Defective transforming
    capacity of adenovirus type 5 host-range mutants, *Virol.*, *86*:10-
    21 (1978).

62. Seif, R., and Martin, R., Growth state of the cell early after
    infection with Simian virus 40 determines whether the maintenance
    of transformation will be A-gene dependent or independent, *J.
    Virol.*, *31*:350-359 (1979).

63. Graessmann, A., Graessman, M., Tjian, R., and Topp, W., Simian
    virus 40 small-t protein is required for loss of actin cable
    networks in rat cells, *J. Virol.*, *33*:1182-1191 (1980).

64. Mackey, J., Wold, W., Rigden, P., and Green, M., Transforming
    region of Group A,B, and C adenoviruses: DNA homology studies
    with twenty-nine human adenovirus serotypes, *J. Virol.*, *29*:1056-
    1064 (1979).

MODULATION OF ADENOVIRUS TRANSFORMATION AND REPLICATION BY CHEMICAL CARCINOGENS AND PHORBOL ESTER TUMOR PROMOTERS

Paul B. Fischer
C. S. H. Young

Department of Microbiology
Cancer Center/Institute of Cancer Research
Columbia University
College of Physicians and Surgeons
New York, New York

I. Bernard Weinstein

Division of Environmental Sciences
Cancer Center/Institute of Cancer Research
Columbia University
College of Physicians and Surgeons
New York, New York

Neil I. Goldstein

Monell Chemical Senses Center
Philadelphia, Pennsylvania

Timothy H. Carter

Department of Biological Sciences
St. John's University
Jamaica, New York

INTRODUCTION

A basic tenet of investigators involved in in vitro studies on cell transformation is that the cellular alterations observed in cells transformed by chemical carcinogens or viruses in vitro may be analogous to neoplastic changes occurring in vivo (for review see 1). Although this concept is probably an over simplification, well defined cell culture systems do represent powerful tools for analyzing the complex multifactorial nature of carcinogenesis without the added

complication of host mediated processes. Carcinogens have been shown
to interact synergistically with various viruses in the development
of neoplasia in vivo and have recently been found to enhance transformation of cells in culture by both DNA and RNA tumor viruses (for review see [2]). In analyzing the synergistic interaction between initiating chemical carcinogens and viruses, a different temporal relationship in the enhancement of viral transformation has been found
for DNA versus RNA tumor viruses. In the case of DNA viruses, such
as adenovirus [3-6] and SV40 [7-9], pretreatment or cotreatment with
specific carcinogens was required for enhancement of viral transformation. This relationship between exposure to the carcinogen and the
virus has been interpreted as an indication that DNA damage and repair
of host cell DNA, which is often associated with exposure to certain
classes of carcinogens, results in an increase in potential viral integration sites in host cell DNA and consequently enhanced viral transformation [4]. In contrast, enhancement of transformation by RNA leukemia virus occurred when carcinogens were applied to previously infected cells [10,11]. The mechanism involved in this synergy is not
known.

The development of an autonomous tumor cell population following
exposure to a carcinogenic agent often involves a series of progressive
alterations in the phenotype of the initiated cells which occurs over
an appreciable portion of the animal's lifespan [1,12]. Studies em-
ploying mouse skin have demonstrated at least two qualitatively different stages in carcinogenesis, one termed "initiation" and the other
"promotion" (for reviews see [13-17]). Unlike initiators which are
carcinogenic, mutagenic, and yield electrophiles which covalently
bind to cell macromolecules, promoters are not "solitary" carcinogens
or mutagenic, and there is no direct evidence that covalent binding
to DNA is required for activity (for reviews see [18-20]). Utilizing
cell culture systems, the most potent tumor promoting agent TPA (12-
0-tetradecanoyl-phorbol-13-acetate) and related plant diterpene esters
have shown to exert a wide range of biological effects including alterations in: cell surface properties; growth properties; and patterns
of differentiation [19-21]. TPA has also recently been shown to

enhance transformation of cell cultures previously exposed to chemical carcinogens [22,23], UV light [24], X-irradiation [25], human adenovirus type 5 [5,6,21], SV40 virus [26], or Epstein-Barr virus [27].

In the present manuscript, we review studies from our laboratories on the effects of chemical carcinogens, tumor promoters and related compounds on: transformation of secondary rat embryo cells (RE) and a cloned population of Fischer rat embryo cells (CREF) by a temperature sensitive mutant of adenovirus type 5 (H5ts125); the expression of transformation associated phenotypes in clones of transformants isolated from solvent or carcinogen pretreated cultures; expression of anchorage-independent growth in H5ts125 transformed RE clones; and adenovirus type 5 replication in HeLa cells.

Carcinogen Enhancement of Adenovirus Transformation

Exposure of tissue culture cells to agents which disrupt the integrity of host cell DNA, such as chemical carcinogens, UV, X-rays or DNA base analogs, as well as agents which do not induce gross alterations in DNA, i.e. tumor promoters and hormones, can result in enhanced SV40 or adenovirus transformation (Table 1) (for review see [2,6]). In previous studies, we have demonstrated that pretreatment of secondary rat embryo (2^ORE) cells with the initiating carcinogens benzo(a)pyrene (BP) or 7,12-dimethylbenz(a)anthracene (DMBA) prior to infection with a temperature-sensitive mutant of type 5 adenovirus (H5ts125) results in a 2- to 4-fold enhancement in viral transformation [5]. Carcinogen induced cytotoxicity was not a prerequisite for this enhancement since an increase in viral transformation resulted even at carcinogen levels which did not induce a reduction in cell cloning efficiency.

In attempting to explain the mechanisms involved in carcinogen enhancement of DNA virus transformation, one could envision at least two possible hypotheses. Carcinogens might enhance viral transformation by: (a) increasing the amount and/or specific region of adenovirus DNA integrated on a per cell basis, thereby increasing the probability of individual cells becoming transformed; or (b) increasing the number of cells in the infected population integrating H5ts125

TABLE 1
Viral Sequences Present in Rat Embryo Cells Transformed by H5ts125
Following Treatment with Benzo(a)pyrene or 7,12-dimethylbenz(a)anthracene

Cell Line[b]	Number of Copies of Hind III Restriction Fragments Present per Diploid Cell Genome[a]						
	G	E	C	D	A	B	F
H5ts125 transformed							
Ad-A18	5.2	5.8	5.5	4.2	3.7	4.7	5.4
Ad-E7	14.6	12.5	1.2	0.2	0	0.05	0.1
Ad-115	20.9	14.3	3.3	0.1	0.06	0.6	3.5
BP pretreated, H5ts125 transformed							
BP-Ad-2	4.0	3.5	0.5	0.2	0.06	0.02	0.5
BP-Ad-E11	1.7	1.3	0.9	1.3	0.7	0.8	1.4
BP-Ad-F1	2.0	3.9	3.1	2.7	1.4	2.1	5.3
BP-Ad-J1	2.4	1.9	1.6	2.9	1.4	0.5	0.6
DMBA pretreated, H5ts125 transformed							
DMBA-Ad-A6	6.7	7.8	3.0	7.1	0.9	0.1	1.2
DMBA-Ad-B8	3.4	3.2	3.0	3.7	2.9	2.5	3.3
DMBA-Ad-C5	2.4	2.4	1.8	1.7	1.5	1.1	0.03

[a]Determined by measuring the reassociation kinetics of excess cellular unlabelled DNA and Ad5 Hind III restriction fragments labelled by nick translation with ^{32}P. Data from H and I are not presented because of the variability of the renaturation kinetics. Further details can be found in Dorsch-Hasler et al. [32].

[b]The origin of these cell lines has been described previously [5,28]. A18 and E7 were obtained following pretreatment of secondary rat embryo ($2^{o}RE$) cells with 0.5% acetone (solvent control); D2, E11 and J1 received 0.05 μg of BP per ml; F1 received 0.5 μg of BP per ml; and A6, B8 and C5 received 0.05 μg of DMBA per ml 18 hours before transformation with the temperature-sensitive mutant of adenovirus type 5 (H5ts125).

Source: Data from [32].

DNA into their cellular genomes, thereby increasing the probability that more cells will become stably transformed. To determine if (a) is the correct hypothesis, we have isolated a series of H5ts125 transformed RE clones from cultures that were pretreated with solvent or carcinogen prior to viral infection [28], and analyzed the quantity

of integrated viral DNA by C_0t analysis [29,30], as well as the state
of integrated viral DNA, by the Southern [31] blotting filter hybridization technique [6,32]. As can be seen in Table 1 carcinogen pretreatment did not alter in any consistent manner either the total quantity or specific regions of H5ts125 DNA that was integrated in the
DNA of these clones. Recent studies by Casto et al. [33] also suggest
that carcinogen pretreatment does not alter the quantity of integrated
simian adenovirus 7 (SA7) DNA in virally transformed hamster embryo
clones. In addition, we have demonstrated using the Southern [31]
blotting filter hybridization technique that carcinogen pretreatment
does not alter the state of integrated viral DNA in transformed clones
[32]. These findings argue against the hypothesis that carcinogen
enhancement of DNA virus transformation results because the DNA damag-
ing agent alters the amount or state of viral DNA integrated in individual transformants. The second hypothesis, that carcinogens increase
the number of cells containing integrated viral DNA, is presently being
evaluated utilizing a recently developed clone of Fischer RE cells
(CREF) which is transformed >150-fold more efficiently than 2^0RE cells
[6,34].

Effects of Carcinogen Pretreatment on the Phenotypic Expression of Transformation Associated Properties in Adenovirus Transformed Rat Embryo Clones

To further explore the role of carcinogens in modulating viral transformation, we have analyzed a spectrum of phenotypic properties in
clones of viral transformants either pretreated with solvent or carcinogen prior to viral infection [28,35]. When contrasted with normal
RE cells, both types of transformed clones generally exhibited a reduction in population doubling time, epidermal growth factor receptors,
serum requirement and cell surface fibronectin; an increase in liquid
cloning efficiency, plasminogen activator production and concanavalin
A agglutinability; and a decrease in anchorage-dependence. No consistent differences were found in these properties when we compared solvent versus carcinogen pretreated H5ts125 transformed H5ts125 transformed clones. However, transformed clones isolated from carcinogen

TABLE 2

Properties of Early Passage Solvent or Carcinogen Pretreated
Adenovirus Transformed Rat Embryo Cells

Cell Type	Agar Cloning Efficiency (%)	Liquid Cloning Efficiency (%)	Fibronectin (% of RE)
Normal			
Secondary rat Embryo (2^0RE)	<.001	3.1	100
Adenovirus-transformed			
Ad-A18	<.001	12.4	75
Ad-B14	<.001	16.2	40
Ad-E7	<.001	4.7	10
Ad-G12	<.01	7.3	32
Benzo(a)pyrene pretreated, adenovirus-transformed			
BP-Ad-D2	0.2	22.6	67
BP-Ad-E11	1.1	33.2	59
BP-Ad-F1	8.5	14.5	80
BP-Ad-J1	2.6	19.2	20
7,12-Dimethylbenz(a)anthracene pretreated, adenovirus-transformed			
DMBA-Ad-A6	3.9	42.2	60
DMBA-Ad-B8	0.8	17.6	36
DMBA-Ad-C5	0.3	9.8	16
DMBA-Ad-H6	1.4	22.5	90

[a]Clones transformed by H5ts125 were isolated from virally infected 2^0RE cultures, derived from 14-day gestation Sprague-Dawley RE's as previously described [5,28]. Some cultures were pretreated with carcinogens (BP, 0.05 µg/ml - D2, E11 and J1; BP, 0.5 µg/ml - F1; or DMBA, 0.05 µg/ml - A6, B8, C5 and H6) prior to virus infection and are so designated. Clones were tested prior to their 20th passage (early passage, -E).

[b]Cells (10^3, 10^4 or 10^5) in low Ca^{2+} medium containing 0.4% Noble agar were layered onto 0.8% agar base layers prepared in the same medium. Colonies >0.2 mm were scored after 21 days. (Further details can be found in [28].

[c]One hundred or 200 H5ts125-transformed 2^0RE cells, or 10^3 2^0RE cells were seeded in low-Ca^{2+} medium (0.1 mM), the medium was changed after 24 hours and thereafter 2 times/week. Colonies >50 cells were enumerated after 2 weeks of growth. (For further details see [28]).

[d]Determination of iodinated fibronectin by SDS-polyacrylamide gel electrophoresis was performed as previously described [28,36]. Values presented are averages from 3 separate samples compared with 2^0RE fibronectin (which was normalized to 100%).

Source: Data from [28].

pretreated cultures did appear to develop anchorage-independence (Table 2) [28], alterations in cell surface glycoprotein profiles [36] and a decreased Ca^{2+} requirement [37] after earlier subpassages than the transformed clones isolated from cultures not exposed to the carcinogen.

Transformation of fibroblast or epithelial cells by chemical carcinogens or viruses has been shown to result in major changes in cell surface composition [36,44,51]. In a number of systems, a direct correlation has been observed between alterations in surface proteins and glycoproteins and the acquisition of anchorage-independent growth [52], as well as in vivo tumorigenicity [49,53]. We have recently analyzed the glycoproteins, glycopeptides and cell surface proteins of normal and cloned populations of early passage solvent and chemical carcinogen-pretreated H5ts125 transformed $2^{o}RE$ cells to determine if any consistent alterations occur in the surface composition of the different cell types [36]. As can be seen in Figure 1, an early passage culture (Ad-A18-E) of H5ts125 transformed RE cells that were not pretreated with carcinogen contained cell surface glycopeptides which were distinguishable from normal $2^{o}RE$ cells, whereas clones derived from RE cultures exposed to both virus and carcinogen contained slightly higher molecular weight, i.e. faster eluting, glucosamine labelled glycopeptides. The magnitude of the change in the latter transformants was not as great as previously observed in Rous sarcoma viurs transformed Syrian hamster embryo cells [48], SV40 transformed 3T3 cells [52], or carcinogen transformed rat liver epithelial cells [47,52], suggesting that this marker is not a sensitive indicator of adenovirus transformation of RE cells. In addition, although all of the H5ts125 transformed $2^{o}RE$ clones tested exhibited a 25 to 90% reduction in fibronectin, the extent of this surface alteration did not correlate with the expression of other transformation-associated phenotypic markers [36].

Recent studies have suggested a positive correlation between tumorigenicity and the presence of an altered plasma membrane glycoprotein of 100,000 daltons (100K) [49]. A similar cell surface glycoprotein modification has been observed in cultured human haemopoietic cell lines, including the promyelocytic leukemia cell line HL-60 [54],

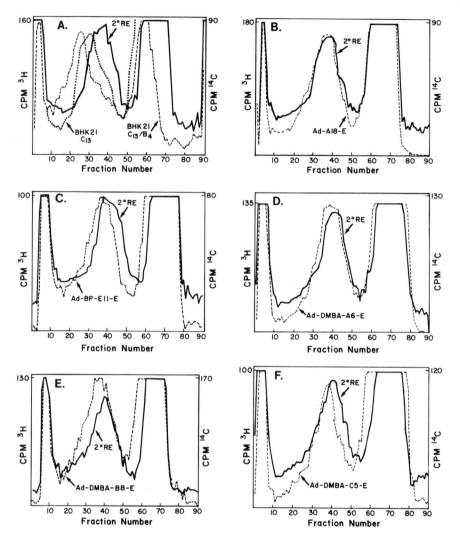

Figure 1. Chromatographic (Sephadex G-50) analysis of glycopeptides from secondary rat embryo (2°RE) cells and solvent- or carcinogen-pretreated adenovirus type 5 (H5ts]25)-transformed RE cells. In all cases the solid line represents the profile of 2°RE cells grown in the presence of ^{14}C-glucosamine and the broken line represents the H5ts]25 transformants grown in ^{3}H-glucosamine. (A) representation of the relative positions of 2°RE (-) and 2 well characterized Syrian hamster lines BHK 2]/C$_{13}$ (....) and BHK 21 C$_{13}$/B$_4$ (---); (B) Ad-A18-E (---) X 2°RE (---); (C) Ad-BP-E11-E (---); X 2°RE (---); (D) Ad-DMBA-A6-E (---); X 2°RE (---); (E) Ad-DMBA-B8-E (---); X 2°RE (---); (F) Ad-DMBA-C5-E (---); X 2°RE (---).
Reprinted with permission from Goldstein and Fisher [36].

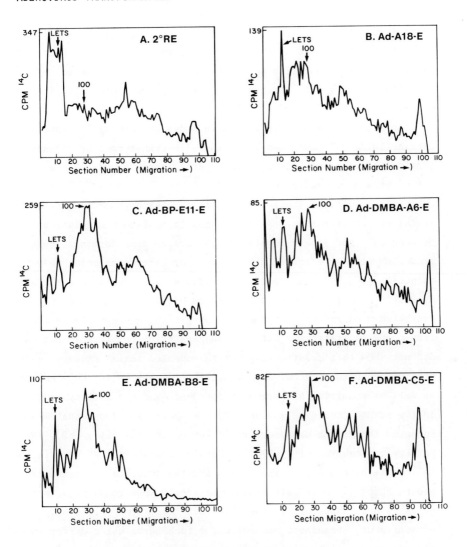

Figure 2. SDS-polyacrylamide gele electrophoresis analysis of cell surface glycoproteins labeled with ^{14}C-glucosamine. For details see Reference 36.
(Reprinted with permission from Goldstein and Fisher [36]).

and certain normal rodent cells treated with TPA (Goldstein and Fisher, unpublished data). We have observed a glycoprotein peak of approximately 100K in a series of early passage H5ts125 transformed clones isolated from RE cultures that had been pretreated with chemical

carcinogens prior to viral infection (Figure 2) [36]. This cell surface component was not as prominent in normal RE or Ad-A18-E cells.
We are presently analyzing additional early and late passage control
RE cultures and various transformed clones to determine its significance.

An altered response to growth in media containing low levels of
extracellular Ca^{2+} has been found in cells transformed by viruses or
chemical carcinogens [55-62]. In general, transformed cells are capable of growing in media containing 0.001 to 0.01 mM Ca^{2+}, whereas under
identical conditions their normal cell counterparts are incapable of
sustained proliferation. We have begun to analyze the relationship
between Ca^{2+} and growth regulation in H5ts125 transformants isolated
from 2°RE cells pretreated with solvent or carcinogen prior to viral
infection [37]. As can be seen in Table 4, when analyzed early after
isolation normal and solvent pretreated H5ts125 transformed RE cells
exhibited a marked Ca^{2+} dependence for growth, whereas clones isolated
from cultures pretreated with carcinogens prior to viral infection
did not show this relationship. With repeated serial passage, solvent-
pretreated cultures acquired the ability to grow in low Ca^{2+} medium
as well as acquiring anchorage-independence and the ability to grow
in low serum containing medium [28]. We have also found that TPA
enhanced the growth of normal rat liver epithelial cells [62], early
passage rat embryo cells [37] and H5ts125 transformed RE [37] in low
Ca^{2+} containing medium. The reason for the lower Ca^{2+} dependence for
growth observed in certain transformed cells when compared with normal
cells is not known. It is possible that transformed cells have: more
effective Ca^{2+} transport mechanisms; mitochondria which differ in Ca^{2+}
sequestering ability; intracellular processes that are less dependent
on Ca^{2+}; or altered Ca^{2+} receptors (such as calmodulin). Since this
phenotype appears to correlate with the development of other properties
associated with the transformed state, an understanding of the mechanism by which cells progress to a state of Ca^{2+} independence may prove
crucial in elucidating the multistep nature of carcinogenesis.

TABLE 4
Effect of Extracellular Ca^{2+} on the Growth of Normal Rat Embryo (RE)
and Early and Late Passage H5ts125 Transformed RE Cells

Cell Type[b]	Pretreatment[c]	Passage Number	Cells per $cm^2 X10^{-4a}$		
			1.25 mM Ca^{2+}	0.01 mM Ca^{2+}	1.25/0.01 Ratio
RE-I	None	5	2.5	0.6	4.2
RE-I$_2$	None	3	3.7	0.6	6.2
RE-I$_3$	None	4	2.9	1.3	2.2
RE-I$_3$	None	20	3.1	1.4	2.2
Ad-A18-E	Acetone	10	10.6	3.4	3.1
Ad-A18-L	Acetone	34	14.5	14.0	1.0
BP-Ad-E11-E	BP	8	14.7	14.8	1.0
BP-Ad-E11-L	BP	45	15.6	15.1	1.0
DMBA-Ad-A6-E	DMBA	10	13.7	13.5	1.0
DMBA-Ad-A6-L	DMBA	29	14.1	14.3	1.0

[a]Five X 10^4 cells were seeded in 5 cm tissue culture dishes, the medium was removed after 24 hours, the cells were washed 2 times with Ca^{2+} and Mg^{2+} free PBS and normal (1.25 mM) or low (0.01 mM) Ca^{2+} was added. Cell counts (4 plates per group) were performed after an additional 5 days and the cell density per replicate plate varied by <10%. For further details see [62].
Source: Data from [37].

[b]I$_1$, I$_2$, and I$_3$ refer to different isolates of pooled populations of 14-day gestation Sprague-Dawley RE's. The three H5ts125 transformed RE clones have been described in Tables 1 and 2. E, early passage, <15 clones; L, later passage, >25, clones.

[c]Ad-A18 cells were pretreated with 0.5% acetone; BP-Ad-E11 cells were pretreated with 0.05 µg of DMBA per ml - prior to transformation with H5ts125.

Enhancement of Adenovirus Transformation
by Tumor Promoters and Related Compounds

The frequency of adenovirus transformation of 2°RE cells [5], and of

a cloned population of Fischer rat embryo (CREF) cells (Table 4) [6,

34], is also enhanced when virally infected cells are grown continuously in TPA. Enhancement of viral transformation by tumor promoters
was observed in both carcinogen- and solvent-pretreated H5ts125 infected 2^0RE cells and appears to involve a selective effect of TPA
on expression of the transformed phenotype [2,5,6,19,28,42,43]. The
ability of tumor promoters to enhance viral transformation is not restricted to adenovirus and rat embryo cells since TPA also enhances
transformation in SV40 virus infected Chinese hamster lung cells [26]
and Epstein-Barr (EB) virus infected human leukocytes [27].

In addition to its effects on viral transformation, tumor promoters have also been shown to induce expression of EB virus and other
oncogenic herpes-viruses in presistently infected cells [63,64], enhance EB virus DNA synthesis [64,65], stimulate the synthesis of mouse
mammary tumor virus (MMTV) in an MMTV producing C3H mouse mammary
tumor cell line [67], and accelerate adenovirus type 5 (Ad5) replication in HeLa cells [68]. The ability of TPA to enhance viral transformation, as well as alter other viral-cell interactions, could result, therefore, from a direct effect of tumor promoters on viral
gene replication and/or expression. We have approached this problem
by analyzing the effect of TPA and related phorbol esters on viral
replication and gene expression during a productive Ad5 infection in
HeLa cells [68]. These studies will be discussed later in this review.

The initial target for TPA action appears to involve the cell
membrane [19,20,69-75]. This concept has been reinforced by recent
studies indicating that the membranes of fibroblast and mouse epidermal
cells contain high affinity saturable receptors for phorbol ester
tumor promoters [74,75]. A relationship between the cell surface and
tumor promoter action is further suggested by the observation that a
membrane active bee venom polypeptide, melittin (MEL), is capable of
inducing cellular effects similar to those of TPA [76]. Treatment
of cells with TPA or MEL results in: (a) an increase in arachidonic
acid and prostaglandin E_2 release from 10T½ cells; (b) an inhibition
in terminal differentiation of mouse B-16 melanoma cells; and (c) enhanced anchorage-independent growth in a clone of H5ts125 transformed
RE cells (E11) [75]. Another polypeptide which initially interacts
with cell surface receptors and induces several biological effects

TABLE 5
Effect of Tumor Promoters and Related Compounds on H5ts125 Transformation
of Clones Fischer Rat Embryo Cells (CREF)

Compound[a]	Concentration	Transformation Foci[b]	Transformation Frequency[c]	Enhancement Factor[d]
Control	DMSO .01%	84+ 6	420	—
	Media	81+ 7	405	—
Phorbol	100 ng/ml	88+11	440	1.1
4-0-meTPA	100 ng/ml	83+ 5	415	1.0
4-α-PDD	100 ng/ml	80+ 9	400	1.0
TPA	100 ng/ml	143+16	715	1.7
TPA	10 ng/ml	135+12	675	1.6
PDD	10 ng/ml	130+10	650	1.6
EGF	10 ng/ml	122+ 8	610	1.5
MEL	2 μg/ml	128+ 9	640	1.6

[a]TPA = 12-0-tetradecanoyl-phorbol-13-acetate; 4αPDD=4α-phorbol-12,13-didecanoate; EGF = epidermal growth factor; MEL = melittin.

[b]One X 10^6 CREF cells were infected with 3 PFU/cell of H5ts125, replated at 2X10^5 cells/ 5cm plate and 72 hours post-infection switched to low Ca^{2+} medium containing the indicated compounds. Plates were fixed after 4 to 5 weeks in formaldehyde and stained with Giemsa solution. Values represent average colony number from 7 plates $\pm$ standard error of the mean.

[c]Number of foci per 10^6 infected cells.

[d]The enhancement factor is the transformation frequency in treated cultures relative to control cultures.
Source: Data from [6] and [90].

that are similar to those of the phorbol esters is epidermal growth
factor (EGF). Both TPA and EGF have been found to induce plasminogen
activator, ornithine decarboxylase and prostaglandin synthesis; stimulate cell growth in both liquid and agar medium; enhance sugar transport; and promote mouse skin tumorigenesis (For review see [20,43]).
These observations prompted us to compare the effects of TPA, MEL and
EGF on adenovirus transformation of CREF cells (Figure 3), (Table 5)
[6,34,90]. All three compounds enhanced H5ts125 transformation, suggesting that alterations in cell membrane function may play an important role in phorbol ester enhancement of viral transformation. These

and related compounds should, therefore, prove extremely valuable for elucidating the mechanisms involved in the action of tumor promoters and for further studies on multifactor interactions in cell transformation.

Modulation of Anchorage-Independent Growth by Tumor Promoters

Of the numerous in vitro parameters which have been evaluated, loss of anchorage-dependence, i.e., growth in agar or agarose suspension, has been found to correlate best with in vivo tumorigenicity [1,38,41]. Although TPA has been shown to induce many changes in normal cells which mimic those observed in cells transformed by chemical carcinogens or viruses, tumor promoters have not been able to induce anchorage-independence in normal cells [18-20]. We have recently demonstrated that TPA and related phorbol ester tumor promoters can induce and enhance agar growth in a series of H5ts125 transformed RE clones (Table 3) [2,6,21,28,42,43]. This effect is not restricted to the adenovirus system since TPA has also recently been shown to enhance anchorage-independence in carcinogen treated mouse epidermal cell cultures [77, 78].

To evaluate the mechanism involved in tumor promoter enhancement of anchorage-independent growth, we utilized a clone of BP pretreated and H5ts125 transformed 2°RE cells, clone E11 [5,28]. Detailed investigations [43] have demonstrated that: (a) incorporation of TPA into the agar medium results in an increase in the number of colonies and they tend to be larger and more diffuse; (b) as little as 1 ng/ml TPA enhances agar growth and maximal enhancement results with 3 ng/ml TPA; and (c) with a series of diterpenes there is a good correlation between tumor promoting activity on mouse skin and enhanced anchorage-independent growth of clone E11 cells. Unlike the majority of TPA effects, which are reversible when the tumor promoter is removed [18-20], the acquisition of anchorage-independence appears to be irreversible since subclones of E11 cells isolated from agar containing TPA subsequently clone 3- to 14-fold more efficiently than the parental cells when re-seeded in agar lacking TPA [2,6,42,43]. It is worth noting that sub-

TABLE 3

Effect of Serial Passage and Exposure to 12-0-tetradecanoyl-phorbol-13-acetate (TPA) on Anchorage-Independent Growth of H5ts125 Transformed Rat Embryo Clones

Cell Type[b]	Agar Cloning Efficiency (%)[a]		Enhancement Factor[c]
	-TPA	+TPA	
Normal			
Secondary rat embryo (2^{O}RE)	< .001	< .001	0
Adenovirus-transformed			
Ad-A18-E	< .001	0.1	> 100
Ad-A18-L	0.1	0.5	5.0
Ad-E7-E	< .001	0.2	> 200
Ad-E7-L	1.2	2.7	2.3
Benzo(a)pyrene pretreated, adenovirus-transformed			
BP-Ad-D2-E	0.2	0.5	2.5
BP-Ad-D2-L	4.1	7.1	1.7
BP-Ad-E11-E	1.1	2.9	2.6
BP-Ad-E11-L	3.0	11.6	3.9
7,12-Dimethylbenz(a)anthracene pretreated, adenovirus-transformed			
DMBA-Ad-A6-E	3.9	6.5	1.7
DMBA-Ad-A6-L	6.7	10.7	1.6
DMBA-Ad-B8-E	0.8	1.3	1.6
DMBA-Ad-B8-L	0.9	1.9	2.0
DMBA-Ad-C5-E	0.3	0.6	2.0
DMBA-Ad-C5-L	0.4	0.7	1.8

[a]The agar cloning assay is described in Table 2 and in detail in [28].

[b]The various cell lines have been described in Tables 1 and 2. E, early passage, < 20 clones; L, later passage, > 25 clones.

[c]The enhancement factor is the agar cloning efficiency in TPA treated relative to solvent (DMSO) treated cultures.
Source: Data from [28].

clones of E11 cells isolated from agar lacking TPA also subsequently demonstrate a 3- to 10-fold enhancement in agar cloning when retested in agar. With 19 of 20 agar-derived subclones, isolated in the presence or absence of TPA, addition of tumor promoters resulted in a further 1.3- to 4.8-fold enhancement in agar growth. These findings

suggest that TPA may be accelerating the expression of a stable phenotype, i.e., anchorage-independence, which develops in certain virally
or chemically transformed cells when they are grown under the selective
pressure of agar.

The ability of tumor promoters to enhance anchorage-independent
growth does not appear to involve random mutation and cell selection
since continued growth of clone E11 cells in liquid medium containing
TPA for 1 month did not result in a population of cells displaying
an enhanced agar growth efficiency in the absence of TPA [43]. Similarly, fluctuation analysis, performed by recloning E11 cells in liquid
medium demonstrated that all of the subclones could grow in agar with
efficiencies of 0.2% to 5.7%, and TPA further enhanced the growth of
the subclones 2.2 to 10-fold. Further evidence for the TPA induction
of the anchorage-independent phenotype was the observation that growth
of specific H5ts125 transformed clones (e.g., A18-E or E7-E), in agar
only occurred if TPA was present in the agar (Table 3). However, when
TPA-induced agar subclones were isolated and retested in agar, they
expressed anchorage-independence in the absence of TPA. Our studies
do not exclude the possibility that TPA also plays a selective role
in this process.

Development of neoplastic potential in BP treated Syrian hamster
embryo cells has been shown to involve a series of progressive alterations in cellular phenotype which occur after repeated subculture
[79,80]. In this system, changes in cell morphology are observed by
8 days post-treatment, fibrinolytic activity appears by 14 days post-
treatment and anchorage-independence and tumorigenicity do not occur
until 6 or more weeks after treatment with BP [79]. Similar changes
in phenotype following repeated subculture have been observed in carcinogen treated guinea pig embryo cells [81], rat brain cells [82],
rat liver cells [83] and mouse epidermal cells [77,78]. Our results
indicate that certain H5ts125 transformed RE clones also undergo a
series of progressive alterations in their phenotype with repeated

serial passage and that this process can be accelerated with TPA [28, 42]. Thus, when studied at early passage, certain H5ts125 transformed RE clones were only capable of growth in agar when TPA was present. With repeated serial passage, however, they spontaneously acquired this phenotype, although TPA could also further enhance agar growth of late passage anchorage-independent clones [2,28]. To investigate the mechanism involved in spontaneous and TPA induced progression in H5ts125 transformed RE clones, we have compared by nucleic acid hybridization the state and pattern of viral DNA integration in the genome of clone E11, after both early (-E) and late (-L) passage, and a series of E11-L subclones isolated from agar containing or lacking TPA and exhibiting a 3- to 14-fold enhanced cloning efficiency in agar [42]. These investigations have demonstrated that: (a) both E11-E and E11-L contain approximately one complete copy of the entire adenovirus type 5 genome; (b) the pattern of viral DNA integration, as indicated by the Southern blotting filter hybridization technique [31], is similar in E11-E and E11-L cells; and (c) the pattern of viral DNA integration in the subclones isolated from agar in the absence or presence of TPA is indistinguishable from the E11-L parental cells.

The mechanism involved in the spontaneous "progression" in the phenotype of adenovirus transformed RE cells, as well as TPA's ability to accelerate this process, is not known. Possible mechanisms include: (a) alterations in the abundance or state of integration of adenovirus sequences; (b) changes in the expression of adenovirus sequences, possibly as a consequence of altered DNA methylation, at the level of transcription and RNA processing or protein synthesis; (c) alterations in the expression of specific host genes which might act in concert with integrated viral genes to modulate this phenotype in the transformants; or (d) karyotype instability which could influence one or more of the former mechanisms. As discussed above, we have obtained evidence that mechanisms (a) does not appear to be the explanation, but the remaining mechanisms require further study.

Alterations in the Temporal Program of Adenovirus Replication
in Human Cells by Tumor Promoters

As previously discussed, TPA has been shown to enhance viral transformation [2,5,26,27] and viral replication [64-66] in a number of
diverse cell culture and virus systems. The ability of tumor promoters
to alter viral-cell interactions may result from a direct or indirect
effect of these agents on viral and/or host genes. In the case of
normal and Rous sarcoma virus-transformed chick embryo fibroblasts,
the addition of TPA results in a profound alteration in cellular phenotype which does not appear to involve an alteration in the level of
protein kinases encoded by the viral src or endogenous sarc genes [85,
86]. To further evaluate the effect of TPA on viral gene expression,
we have analyzed the effect of tumor promoters on the kinetics of
Ad5 replication in human cells. We found that the addition of TPA
at the time of infection, or up to 8 hours post-infection, accelerates
the appearance of early virus antigens (72K DNA-binding protein), the
onset of viral DNA synthesis and the production of infectious virus
(Figure 4). TPA and related phorbol esters, but not structurally similar compounds inactive as tumor promoters on mouse skin [13-17] (i.e.,
phorbol and 4αphorbol-12,13-didecanoate), also induced a dramatic
early cytopathic effect (CPE) in infected HeLa cultures (Figure 5).
The morphology change in infected cells did not result from a sensiti-
zation of cells to the effects of viral antigens or the induction of
plasminogen activator [84]. Analysis of viral mRNA synthesis did
indicate, however, that tPA accelerated the production of mRNA from
all major early regions, transiently stimulated region III mRNA approximately 3-fold and accelerated the appearance of late mRNA (Figures
6 and 7). There is also evidence that TPA can alter the production
of discrete classes of mRNA in normal and tumorigenic cells [67,89].
These studies indicate that nPA has a primary and early effect on Ad5
replication in permissive human cells and that this effect involves
viral mRNA production.

The TPA induced morphology change in uninfected HeLa cells and
the accelerated CPE in Ad5 infected cells was not blocked by addition

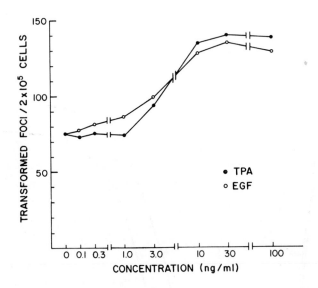

Figure 3. Dose-response to TPA and epidermal growth factor (EGF) of adenovirus transformation of CREF cells. Transformation assays using CREF cells and H5ts125 were performed as described in Table 5 using 10 plates per point. Values represent average number of foci per plate, replicates varied by <15%, ●—●, TPA, o—o, EGF.

or leupeptin, antipain or trans-retinoic acid. The TPA induced alterations in uninfected HeLa cells may involve changes in the cytoskeleton,
since TPA has been shown to induce such modifications in chick embryo
fibroblast cells and this effect also is not blocked by protease inhibitors [87]. As mentioned above, in the case of Ad5 infected cells,
the TPA enhancement of CPE could be due to an acceleration of the viral
replicative cycle (Figure 3). In addition, hybridization results
demonstrate that production of virus mRNA is dramatically affected
by exposure of cells to nanogram quantities of TPA at the time of
viral infection (Figures 6 and 7). The accelerated CPE induced by
TPA might also result from the over production of functional region
III mRNA, which encodes a surface glycoprotein associated with the
cytoskeleton [88]. Studies are presently in progress to directly define the mechanism(s) by which TPA induces morphological alterations
in uninfected HeLa cells and accelerates the development of a CPE in
Ad5 infected human cells.

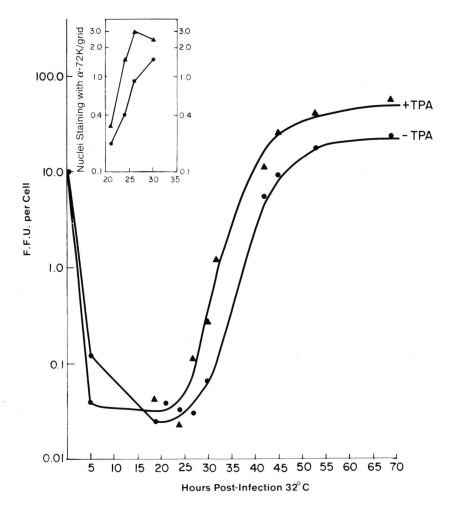

Figure 4. Growth curve of adenovirus type 5 (Ad5) in HeLa cell monolayers and the presence of 72K DNA binding protein in the presence
or absence of TPA. Replicate dishes of HeLa cells were infected with
Ad5 at a multiplicity of infection (m.o.i.) of ∿10 f.f.u./cell. After
2 hour adsorption they were overlaid with growth medium containing
100 ng/ml of TPA. At intervals, dishes were frozen and total virus
was assayed by an indirect fluorescent focus assay. For measurement
of Ad DNA-binding protein (DBP), HeLa cells on glass coverslips were
infected with virus at a m.o.i. of 0.2 f.f.u./cell, and overlaid as
above. At intervals, coverslips were removed, the cells fixed by
air-drying and acetone treatment and the 72K DBP visualized using an
indirect fluorescence technique with rabbit ∝DBP (a gift of Dr. H. S.
Ginsberg [91]).

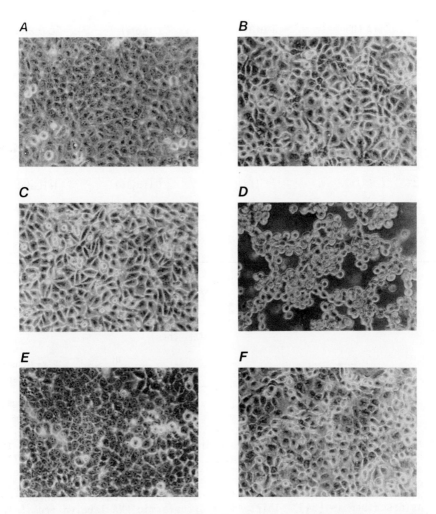

Figure 5. Effect of TPA and phorbol on the morphology of uninfected and adenovirus type 5 (Ad5) infected HeLa cells. Cells were seeded in 35 mm tissue culture dishes at 32°, mock infected or infected with 10 PFU/cell of Ad5, 16 hours post-infection, the various compounds were added and the plates were grown at 39°C for 24 hours and photographed using phase-contrast optics (~150X magnification). (A) Mock-infected; (B) Ad5 infected; (C) Mock-infected cells grown in 100 ng/ml TPA for 24 hours; (D) Ad5 infected cells grown in 100 ng/ml TPA for 24 hours; (E) Mock-infected cells grown in 200 ng/ml phorbol for 24 hours; (F) Ad5 infected cells grown in 200 ng/ml phorbol for 24 hours.

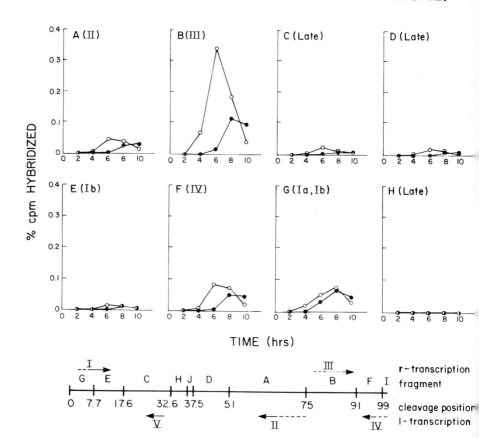

TIME (hrs)

Figure 6. Effect of TPA on adenovirus (Ad5) poly (A) + RNA (2 to 10 h.p. h.p.i.). Confluent HeLa monolayers were infected with 100 PFU/cell Ad5 at 32°C. At intervals 50 μCi/ml ^{3}H-uridine (80 μCi/mmole, NEN) was added and incubation continued for 2 hours. Cytoplasmic poly (A) + RNA was isolated by phenol extraction and oligo (dT) cellulose chromatography as described in [84]. Thirty % of cytoplasmic RNA labeled from 5 to 7 h.p.i. was retained on the column; the % of poly (A) + RNA at each time did not differ significantly in TPA-treated and control cultures. Specific activity on the poly (A) + RNA was 3 to 4 X 10^4 c.p.m./μg. Poly (A) + RNA was hybridized to separated Hind III restriction endonuclease fragments of Ad5 DNA bound to nitrocellulose filters (2.5 μg equivalent per filter). Hybridization is expressed as % of total c.p.m. in the hybridization reaction bound to the filter. Each point on the graph denotes the midpoint of a 2 hour labeling period. The lower figure shows the location of early mRNA on the Ad5 Hind III restriction endonuclease cleavage map. Fragments are designated by letter assigned in order of decreasing size. Map positions are shown as % of the genome length, the positions of major early mRNA groups are indicated by arrows identified by roman numerals.

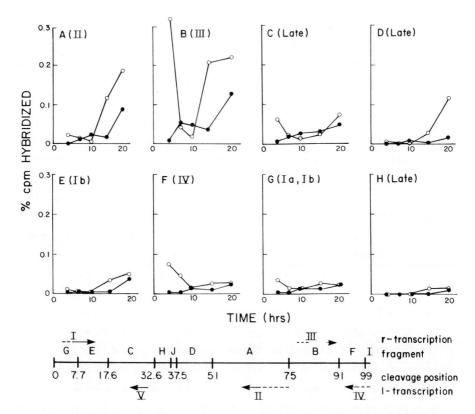

Figure 7. Effect of TPA on adenovirus (Ad5) poly (A) + RNA (4 to 20 h.p.i.). Refer to Figure 6 for experimental details.

SUMMARY

Well characterized cell culture systems are now available for investigating the interactions between initiating chemical carcinogens, tumor promoters and viruses in mammalian cell transformation. We have demonstrated that chemical carcinogens and tumor promoters can enhance the frequency by which a human virus, adenovirus type 5, transforms rat embryo cells. The ability of carcinogens to enhance viral transformation appears to involve an interaction between the metabolically activated carcinogen and cellular DNA. Tumor promoters, in contrast to initiating chemical carcinogens, do not induce DNA damage or repair.

Their ability to enhance viral transformation may result because these compounds alter the program of virus and/or host gene expression involved in transformation. The existence of specific membrane-associated receptors for the tumor promoter TPA, and the fact that the earliest responses of cells to TPA involves alterations in membrane structure and function, suggest that these changes in gene expression may result from TPA induced cell surface modifications. Somewhat similar cell surface modifications might also play a role in subsequent maintenance of the transformed phenotype.

In addition to being multifactor in terms of its etiology, the carcinogenic process also appears to involve several discrete steps in its development. Analysis of individual adenovirus transformed clones indicate that the development of various transformation-associated phenotypes often involves a multistep, progressive process. Initial studies indicate that spontaneous or TPA-enhanced progression in various adenovirus transformed clones, as indicated by an increase in anchorage-independence, does not involve an alteration in the quantity or state of adenovirus DNA integrated into the host cell genome. By generating a family of subclones which vary in their expression of anchorage-independence, i.e., from negligible or no growth in agar to a high agar cloning changes in chromosomal composition or viral gene expression (at the level of RNA transcription and processing or protein synthesis).

Our inability to directly demonstrate a viral etiology for the majority of human neoplasias may be a consequence of the fact that the putative virus induces cancer via synergistic interactions with chemical carcinogens, tumor promoters, hormones or other cofactors. In some forms of cancer, the viral genetic information that initially contribute to the transformation process might ultimately be lost from the human cancer cells, explaining the reason for our inability to detect its presence in the cellular genome by molecular hybridization techniques, as the tumor cell progresses in its development. The inability to investigate potential synergistic relationships between environmental chemicals and viruses at a molecular level in controlled cell culture systems should, therefore, provide valuable information on the role of these agents in the etiology of certain human cancers.

ACKNOWLEDGMENTS

The authors are indebted to Drs. Harold S. Ginsberg and Karoline Dorsch-Hasler for their valuable collaboration in several studies described in this paper. The excellent technical assistance of Janet H. Bozzone, Patricia Munz and Eleanor Yee is appreciated. We also thank Patricia Vickman for valuable assistance in preparing this manuscript. This research was supported by grants from the American Cancer Society, RD-50, National Institutes of Health AI-15451, CA-25757 and CA-26056.

REFERENCES

1. Fisher, P. B., and Weinstein, I. B., In vitro screening tests for potential carcinogens. In: Carcinogens in Industry and the Environment, (J. M. Sontag, ed.), Marcel Dekker, New York, 1980, Ch. 6, pp. 113-166.

2. Fisher, P. B., and Weinstein, I. B., Chemical-viral interactions and multistep aspects of cell transformation. In: Molecular and Cellular Aspects of Carcinogen Screening Tests, (R. Montesano, H. Bartsch and L. Tomatis, eds.), IARC Scientific Pub., No. 27, Lyon, France, 1980, pp. 113-131.

3. Casto, B. C., Cancer Res., 33:402-407 (1973).

4. Casto, B. C., Pieczynski, W. J., Janosko, N., and DiPaolo, J. A., Chem.-Biol. Interact., 13:105-125 (1976).

5. Fisher, P. B., Weinstein, I. B., Eisenberg, D., and Ginsberg, H. S., Proc. Natl. Acad. Sci., U.S.A., 75:2311-2314 (1978).

6. Fisher, P. B., Dorsch-Hasler, K., Weinstein, I. B. and Ginsberg, H. S., Teratogenesis, Carcinogenesis and Mutagenesis, 1981, in press.

7. Diamond, L., Knorr, R., and Shimizu, Y., Cancer Res., 34:2599-2604 (1974).

8. Hirai, K., Defendi, V., and Diamond, L., Cancer Res., 34:3497-3500 (1974).

9. Milo, G. E., Blakeslee, J. R., Hart, R., and Yohn, D. S., Chem.-Biol. Interact., 22:185-197 (1978).

10. Price, P. J., Freeman, A. E., Lane, W. T., and Huebner, R. J.,
     Nature-New. Biol., *230:*144-145 (1971).

11. Rhim, J. S., Vass, W., Cho, H. Y., and Huebner, R. J., *Int. J.
     Cancer,* *7:*65-74 (1971).

12. Foulds, L., Neoplastic Development, Vol. 1, Academic Press, New
     York (1969).

13. Van Duuren, B. L., *Prog. Exp. Tumor Res.*, *11:*31-68 (1969).

14. Boutwell, R. K., *CRC Crit. Rev. Toxicol.*, *2:*419-443 (1974).

15. Berenblum, I., Origin of the concept of sequential stages of skin
     carcinogenesis. In: Cancer I (F. F. Becker, ed.), Plenum Pub.
     Corp., New York, 1975, pp. 323-344.

16. Hecker, E., Cocarcinogens and cocarcinogenesis. In: Handbuch
     der Allgemeinen Pathologie (E. Grundman, ed.), IV, Vol. 16,
     Springer-Verlag, Berlin, 1975, pp. 651-676.

17. Slaga, T. J., Sivak, A., and Boutwell, R. K., Mechanisms of Tumor
     Promotion and Cocarcinogenesis, Carcinogenesis Vol. 2, Raven
     Press, New York (1978).

18. Weinstein, I. B., Wigler, M., Fisher, P. B., Sisskin, E., and
     Pietropaolo, C., Cell culture studies on the biological effects
     of tumor promoters. In: Mechanisms of Tumor Promotion and Co-
     carcinogenesis, Carcinogenesis, Vol. 2 (T. J. Slaga, A Sivak,
     and R. K. Boutwell, eds.), Raven Press, New York, 1978, pp. 313-
     333.

19. Weinstein, I. B., Wigler, M., Yamasaki, H., Lee, L. S., Fisher,
     P. B., and Mufson, R. A., Regulation of the expression of certain
     biologic markers of neoplasia. In: Biological Markers of Neo-
     plasia: Basic and Applied Aspects (R. W. Ruddon, ed.), Elsevier
     North-Holland, New York, 1978, pp. 451-471.

20. Weinstein, I. B., Lee, L. S., Fisher, P. B., Mufson, R. A., and
     Yamasaki, H., *J. Supramolecular Struct.*, *12:*195-208 (1979).

21. Fisher, P. B., Guidelines to Metabolic Therapy, 1981, in press.

22. Lasne, C., Gentil, A., and Chouroulinkov, I., *Nature, 247:*490-491
     (1974).

23. Mondal, S., Brankow, D. W., and Heidelberger, C., *Cancer Res.,
     36:*2254-2260 (1976).

24. Mondal, S., and Heidelberger, C., *Nature, 260:*710-711 (1976).

25. Kennedy, A., Mondal, S., Heidelberger, C., and Little, J. B., *Cancer Res.*, *38*:439-443 (1978).

26. Martin, R. G., Setlow, V. P., Edwards, C. A. and Vembu, D., *Cell*, *17*:635-643 (1979).

27. Yamamoto, N., and zur Hausen, H., *Nature*, *280*:244-245 (1979).

28. Fisher, P. B., Goldstein, N. I., and Weinstein, I. B., *Cancer Res.*, *39*:3051-3057 (1979).

29. Britten, R. J., and Kohne, D. K., *Science*, *161*:529-540 (1968).

30. Gallimore, P. H., Sharp, P. A., and Sambrook, J., *J. Mol. Biol.*, *89*:49-72 (1974).

31. Southern, E. M., *J. Mol. Biol.*, *98*:503-517 (1975).

32. Dorsch-Hasler, K., Fisher, P. B., Weinstein, I. B., and Ginsberg, H. S., *J. Virol.*, *34*:305-314 (1980).

33. Casto, B. C., Miyagi, M., Meyers, J., and DiPaolo, J. A., *Chem.-Biol. Interact.*, *25*:255-269 (1979).

34. Fisher, P. B., Mufson, R. A., and Weinstein, I. B., *J. Cell Biol. (Abst.)*, *83*:459 (1979).

35. Fisher, P. B., Lee, L. S., and Weinstein, I. B., *Biochem. Biophys. Res. Commun.*, *93*:1160-1166 (1980).

36. Goldstein, N. I., and Fisher, P. B., *J. Cell Sci.*, in press (1980).

37. Fisher, P. B., and Weinstein, I. B., Carcinogenesis, in submission (1980).

38. Freedman, V. H., and Shin, S., *Cell*, *3*:355-359 (1974).

39. Shin, S., Freedman, V. H., Risser, R., and Pollack, R., *Proc. Acad. Sci.*, *U.S.A.*, *72*:4435-4439 (1975).

40. Weinstein, I. B., Wigler, M., and Stadler, U., Analysis of the mechanism of chemical carcinogenesis in epithelial cell cultures. In: Screening Tests in Chemical Carcinogenesis, (R. Montesano, H. Bartsch, and L. Tomatis, eds.), IARC Scientific Pub., No. 12, Lyon, France, 1976, pp. 355-381.

41. Montesano, R., Drevon, C., Kuroki, T., Saint Vincent, L., Handleman, S., Sanford, K. K., DeFeo, D., and Weinstein, I. B., *J. Natl. Cancer Inst.*, *59*:1651-1658 (1977).

42. Fisher, P. B., Dorsch-Hasler, K., Weinstein, I. B., and Ginsberg, H. S., *Nature*, *281*:591-594 (1979).

43. Fisher, P. B., Bozzone, J. H., and Weinstein, I. B., *Cell, 18:*695-705 (1979).

44. Hynes, R. O., *Proc. Natl. Acad. Sci., U.S.A., 70:*3170-3174 (1973).

45. Hynes, R. O., *Biochim. Biophys. Acta, 458:*73-107 (1976).

46. Pietropaolo, C., Yamaguchi, N., Weinstein, I. B., and Glick, M. C., *Int. J. Cancer, 120:*738-747 (1977).

47. Vaheri, A., and Mosher, D. F., *Biochim. Biophys. Acta, 516:*1-25 (1978).

48. Warren, L., Buck, C. A., and Tuszynski, G. P., *Biochim. Biophys. Acta, 516:*97-127 (1978).

49. Bramwell, M. E., and Harris, H., *Proc. R. Soc. B, 201:*87-106 (1978).

50. Lage-Davila, A., Kurst, B., Hofmann-Clerc, F., Torpier, G., and Montagnier, L., *J. Cell. Physiol., 100:*95-108 (1979).

51. Goldstein, N. I., and Fisher, P. B., *J. Natl. Cancer Inst.,* in press (1981).

52. Smets, L. A., Van Beek, W. P., Van Rooy, H., and Homburg, C. H., *Cancer Biochem. Biophys., 2:*203-207 (1978).

53. Glick, M. C., Rabinowitz, Z., and Sachs, L., *J. Virol., 13:*967-974 (1974).

54. Omary, M. B., Trowbridge, I. S., and Minowada, J., *Nature, 286:*888-891 (1980).

55. Boynton, A. L., and Whitfield, J. F., *Proc. Natl. Acad. Sci., U.S.A., 73:*1651-1654 (1976).

56. Boynton, A. L., and Whitfield, J. F., *Cancer Res., 38:*1237-1240 (1978).

57. Swierenga, S. H. H., Whitfield, J. F., and Gillan, D. J., *J. Natl. Cancer Inst., 57:*125-129 (1976).

58. Swierenga, S. H. H., Whitfield, J. F., and Karasaki, S., *Proc. Natl. Acad. Sci., U.S.A., 75:*6069-6072 (1978).

59. Boynton, A. L., Whitfield, J. F., Isaacs, R. J., and Trembley, R. G., *Cancer Res., 37:*2657-2661 (1977).

60. Boynton, A. L., Whitfield, J. F., Isaacs, R. J., and Trembley, R. G., *J. Cell. Physiol., 92:*241-248 (1977).

61. McKeehan, W. L., and Ham, R. G., *Nature, 275:*756-758 (1978).

62. Fisher, P. B., and Weinstein, I. B., *Cancer Lett., 10:*7-17 (1980).

63. zur Hausen, H., O'Neill, F. J., and Freese, U. K., *Nature, 272:*
    373-375 (1978).

64. zur Hausen, H., Bornkamm, G. W., Schmidt, R., and Hecker, E.,
    *Proc. Natl. Acad. Sci., U.S.A., 76:*782-785 (1979).

65. Lin, J. C., Shaw, J. E., Smith, M. C., and Pagano, J. S., *Virology,*
    *99:*183-187 (1979).

66. Hudewentz, J., Bornkamm, G. W., and zur Hausen, H., *Virology,*
    *100:*175-178 (1980).

67. Arya, S. K., *Nature, 284:*71-72 (1980).

68. Fisher, P. B., Young, C. S. H., Weinstein, I. B., and Carter,
    T. H., *Am. Soc. Microbiol. (Abst.)* (1980).

69. Sivak, A., *J. Cell Physiol., 80:*167-174 (1972).

70. Blumberg, P. M., Driedger, P. E., and Rossow, P. W., *Nature,*
    *264:*446-447 (1976).

71. Driedger, P. E., and Blumberg, P. M., *Cancer Res., 37:*3257-3265
    (1977).

72. Fisher, P. B., Flamm, M., Schachter, D., and Weinstein, I. B.,
    *Biochem. Biophys. Res. Commun., 86:*1063-1068 (1979).

73. Nagle, D. S., and Blumberg, P. M., *Cancer Res., 40:*1066-1072
    (1980).

74. Driedger, P. E., and Blumberg, P. M., *Proc. Natl. Acad. Sci.,*
    *U.S.A., 77:*567-571 (1980).

75. Weinstein, I. B., Mufson, R. A., Lee, L. S., Fisher, P. B.,
    Laskin, J., Horowitz, A. D., and Ivanovic, V., Membrane and other
    biochemical effects of the phorbol esters and their relevance
    to tumor promotion. In: Carcinogenesis: Fundamental Mechanisms
    and Environmental Effects, (B. Pullman, P. O. P. Ts'o, and H.
    Gelboin, eds.), R. Reidel Publ. Co., Amsterdam, Holland, 1980,
    in press.

76. Mufson, R. A., Laskin, J. D., Fisher, P. B., and Weinstein, I. B.,
    *Nature, 280:*72-74 (1979).

77. Colburn, N. H., Vorder Bruegge, W. F., Bates, J. R., Gray, R. H.,
    Rossen, J. D., Kelsey, W. H., and Shimada, T., *Cancer Res., 38:*
    624-634 (1978).

78. Colburn, N. H., Former, B. F., Nelson, K. A., and Yuspa, S. H.,
     Nature, 281:589-591 (1979).

79. Barrett, J. C., Crawford, B. D., Grady, D. L., Hester, L. D.,
     Jones, P. A., Benedict, W. F., and Ts'o, P. O. P., *Cancer Res.,
     37*:3815-3823 (1977).

80. Barrett, J. C., and Ts'o, P. O. P., *Proc. Natl. Acad. Sci., U.S.A.,
     75*:3761-3765 (1978).

81. Evans, C. H., Rabin, E. S., and DiPaolo, J. A., *Cancer Res., 37*:
     898-903 (1977).

82. Laerum, O. D., and Rajewsky, M. J., *J. Natl. Cancer Inst., 55*:
     1177-1187 (1975).

83. Montesano, R., Saint-Vincent, L., and Tomatis, L., *Br. J. Cancer,
     28*:215-220 (1973).

84. Fisher, P. B., Young, C. S. H., Weinstein, I. B., and Carter,
     T. H., manuscript in preparation (1980).

85. Goldberg, A. R., Delclos, K. B., and Blumberg, P. M., *Science,
     208*:191-193 (1980).

86. Laskin, J. D., Pietropaolo, C., Erikson, R. L. and Weinstein,
     I. B., Abstract to AACR, San Diego, Calif., 1980.

87. Rifkin, D. B., Crowe, R. M. and Pollack, R., *Cell, 18*:361-368
     (1979).

88. Ross, S. and Levine, A. J., *Virology, 99*:427-430 (1979).

89. Gottesman, M. M., and Sobel, M. E., *Cell, 19*:449-455 (1980).

90. Fisher, P. B., Mufson, R. A., Weinstein, I. B., and Little, J. B.,
     manuscript in preparation (1980).

91. Ginsberg, H. S., Lundholm, U. and Linne, T., *J. Virol., 23*:142-
     151 (1977).

TRANSFORMATION OF MURINE FIBROBLASTS BY NORMAL MOUSE CELL DNA FRAGMENTS: POSSIBLE IMPLICATIONS FOR MODELS OF NONVIRAL CARCINOGENESIS

K. J. van den Berg
V. Krump-Konvalinkova
P. A. Bentvelzen
D. W. van Bekkum

Radiobiological Institute TNO
Rijswijk
The Netherlands

INTRODUCTION

Tumor virological studies continue to be of general interest, because they provide experimental approaches for unravelling the process of neoplastic transformation, not only by oncogenic viruses but also by other agents. A common step between viral carcinogenesis and radiation or chemical carcinogenesis could be a somatic mutation of the cellular genetic material. The mutation in the case of virally induced transformation, however, is a very special one. It involves the insertion of a specific transforming gene(s) (onc gene) into the cellular genome at many different sites. This often leads to a continuous production of transforming proteins which, depending on the epigenetic status of the cell, may result in oncogenic conversion.

The onc-genes of so-called rapidly transforming RNA tumor viruses
seem to be derived from cellular genetic material [1-9]. It has been
postulated that, during the complicated recombination process which
generated these highly oncogenic viruses, modification of these cellular genes bestowing oncogenic potential on them has occurred [10].
This latter idea would be comparable to the simplistic somatic mutation
hypothesis in nonviral carcinogenesis, invoking a point mutation leading to an altered gene-product with such different physiological properties that neoplastic conversion would result.

A more attractive, less complicated assumption is that rapid viral
transformation is due to the introduction of an unmodified cellular
gene controlling growth and/or differentiation into a different site
of the cellular genome. Associated viral promotor sequences would
cause overproduction of a polypeptide regulating growth and/or differentiation. The latter model has different consequences for theories
about radiation and chemical carcinogenesis.

In transfection studies using DNA from various murine cell lines,
Shih et al. [11] found that exposure of normal cells to DNA from chemically transformed cell lines resulted in the production of foci of
transformed cells. Only very rarely could normal cellular DNA transform cells in vitro. These results are compatible with a simple somatic mutation hypothesis. However, Cooper et al. [12] consistently
observed that when sheared mechanically into relatively small fragments,
DNA isolated from normal tissue culture cells induced transformation,
although at a low frequency. Subsequent transfection with DNA, isolated from the transformants resulted in a greatly increased transformation rate when high molecular weight DNA was used.

In the course of our studies on transfection with the provirus
of Abelson murine leukemia virus (A-MuLV), we independently from Cooper
et al. [12] observed that DNA isolated from normal BALB/c mouse thymus
cells could transform fibroblast cell lines. This observation was
then extended to some other tissues of germfree mice. In addition,
we found that preinfection of the recipient cells with murine leukemia
virus resulted in a strong enhancement of transformation by normal
cell DNA fragments.

MATERIALS AND METHODS

Tissue Culture

All cell lines were grown in Dulbecco MEM supplemented with 10% newborn
calf serum. BALB/3T3 and NIH/3T3 cells were used for the various
transformation assays. At various culture passages after treatment
with preparations to be tested for transforming activity, some dishes
were not trypsinized and were examined regularly for 2 weeks for the
appearance of foci of transformed cells. A NIH/3T3 clone chronically
infected with Moloney murine leukemia virus (Mo-MuLV) was kindly provided by Prof. Dr. H. P. J. Bloemers of the University of Nijmegen.
A BALB/3T3 subline infected with Rauscher murine leukemia virus (R-
MuLV) was freshly prepared.

In immunofluorescence studies a battery of cell lines routinely
used in various investigations in our laboratory was tested to determine the specificity of the antisera. This battery includes the lines
mentioned above, a BALB/3T3 subline transformed by A-MuLV, a nonproducer BALB/3T3 line transformed by Abelson proviral DNA, the mouse mammary tumor cell lines C3HMT/c111 and Mm5mt/c1, the normal mouse mammary gland lines C3HMK/Rij and BMK/A, the feline cell line CrFK and
its subline infected with the murine mammary tumor virus (MuMTV).

Transfection

DNA was extracted from tissues of germfree BALB/c mice as follows: A
single cell suspension was made in TNE buffer (10 mM Tris-HCl, pH 7.6,
100 mM NaCl, 1 mM EDTA) and then lysed by the addition of Sarkosyl
to a concentration of 2% and Proteinase K (200 µg. ml^{-1} final concentration) for 16 h at 37°C. The viscous lysate was extracted twice
with an equal volume of phenol-chloroform (1:2 v/v). The viscous upper
layer was then dialyzed for 5 days against 0.1x SSC. The still viscous
solution was incubated with 100 µg. ml^{-1} RNase A for 2 h at 37°C and
then with 100 µg. ml^{-1} pronase for 2 h at 37°C. The resulting solution
was extracted with phenol-chloroform, and then exhaustively dialyzed

against 0.1 x SSC. The DNA was diluted in the so-called transfection
buffer (pH 6.95) of Graham and Van der Eb [13] to a concentration of
50 ug. ml^{-1}, sheared to an average size of about $10x10^6$ daltons by
passing it 29 times through a 0.8 mm syringe needle and precipitated
with 2.5 M $CaCl_2$ to a final concentration of 125 mM. Following this,
0.5 ml of the precipitate was added to 2.5 ml of fresh tissue culture
medium and placed on dishes of 3T3 cells seeded 20 h earlier. Eighteen
hours later, the cells were trypsinized and then subcultured according
to the 3T3 scheme. Focus formation was scored during 2 weeks in a
number of dishes set aside after each subcultivation.

Immunofluorescence

C57BL/Ka mice were immunized with lethally irradiated (20 Gy) syngeneic
A-MuLV-induced lymphoma cells. After the last of 12 i.p. injections
with 10^7 cells at weekly intervals, the mice were bled a week later.
The antiserum was absorbed twice with syngeneic Mo-MuLV-induced lym-
phoma cells. A control antiserum was raised in C3Hf mice against the
MuMTV-S induced mammary tumor cell line C3HMT/c111 [14]. These mice
were subjected to the same immunization scheme as was used for the
A-MuLV-lymphoma cells. The antiserum was absorbed twice with purified
MuMTV-S and with BALB/3T3 cells nonproductively transformed by Moloney
murine sarcoma virus (S^+L^- cells).

After trypsinization of cultured cells, they were deposited on
microscope slides and incubated for 16-20 h in a humidified incubator
(5% CO_2) at 37°C. The cells were then washed 3 x 10 minutes with PBS
and fixed for 3 x 5 minutes in acetone at -28°C. Fixed cells were
washed 2 x 10 minutes in PBS. They were then incubated with 10-, 20-
and 40-fold dilutions of the antiserum for 45 min at room temperature.
After washing 2 x 10 minutes with PBS, the cells were incubated with
goat antiserum to mouse immunoglobulins conjugated with fluorescein
isothiocyanate (Nordic, Tilburg, The Netherlands) diluted 1 : 20 in
PBS. After washing 2 x 10 minutes with PBS, the cells were embedded
in Elvanol. Normal C57BL/Ka mouse serum or only the goat-anti-mouse
serum was included as controls. The embedded cells were examined with

Tumor Bioassay

After trypsinization and washing, approximately 10^6 cells were inoculated intraperitoneally into adult athymic nude mice (with a BALB/c genetic background) or newborn (BALB/c x DBA/2)F1 mice or subcutaneously into 3 week-old BALB/c mice.

RESULTS

The production of foci of transformed cells in dishes of 3T3 cells exposed to DNA isolated from the thymus of germfree BALB/c mice is presented in Table 1. All dishes incubated with normal cell DNA contained such foci. In the BALB/3T3 line the average number of foci per dish was fifteen, in the NIH/3T3 line only four.

Treatment of the DNa fragments with DNase completely abolished their transforming capacity, while RNase or pronase did not. This indicate that transformation can be solely attributed to DNA. Heat denaturation of the DNA resulted in partial abrogation of transforming ability. Neither calf thymus DNA nor E. coli DNA induced foci in either kind of 3T3 cells.

While foci or transformed cells appeared within two weeks after a single passage in our studies on the A-MuLV provirus, the cultures exposed to normal cellular DNA yielded foci later, namely after about six passages performed in the course of one month. In the BALB/3T3 cell line these foci grew in multilayers, while in the NIH/3T3 line foci consisted of rounded, highly refractile cells growing in mono- or bilayers.

DNA isolated from thymus, spleen or liver of germfree BALB/c mice did not differ in transforming capacity (Table 2) indicating that the transforming sequences are present in their germ line and are not due to a recent horizontal infection.

A series of cloned cell lines was developed from BALB/3T3 cells transformed by normal cell DNA. All of these grew well in soft agar. They showed no reverse transcriptase activity with the highly sensitive technique of Aboud et al. [15] was used. No transforming virus

TABLE 1
Transformation of 3T3 Cells by Normal BALB/c DNA

| | Recipient Cells | | | |
| | BALB/3T3 | | NIH/3T3 | |
	Fraction Transformed Cultures	Average No. Foci/Dish	Fraction Transformed Cultures	Average No. Foci/Dish
BALB/c thymus DNA 50 mg.ml^{-1}	16/16	15	16/16	4
Treated with Pronase[a]	8/8	4	7/8	1.5
Treated with RNase[a]	8/8	2	8/8	6
Treated with DNase[a]	0/8	0	0/8	0
Heat denatured[b]	3/8	0.5	3/8	0.5
Calf thymus DNA, 50 μg.ml^{-1}	0/8	0	0/8	0
E. coli DNA, 50 mg.ml^{-1}	0/8	0	0/8	0

[a] 1 hr at 37°C.
[b] 5 min at 100°C, then quickly placed in ice.

TABLE 2
Effect of Origin of BALB/c DNA on Transforming Activity

| | Recipient Cells (Fraction Transformed Cultures) | |
	BALB/3T3	NIH/3T3
Thymus 50 μg.ml^{-1}	16/16	16/16
25 μg.ml^{-1}	8/8	N.D.[a]
Spleen 50 μg.ml^{-1}	8/8	N.D.
25 μg.ml^{-1}	8/8	2/8
Liver 50 μg.ml^{-1}	4/4	N.D.

[a]N.D. = not done.

could be rescued after infection with Mo-MuLV, while such a virus could be readily rescued from lines transformed by DNA isolated from A-MuLV-induced lymphoma cells.

An attempt was made to characterize the products of the transforming genes present in the donor DNA isolated from normal cells. Therefore was employed immunofluorescence with antisera directed against the products of the onc-genes of murine RNA tumor viruses. We had available an antiserum against the nonstructural protein of A-MuLV (see [16]) and against the products of the presumed onc-gene of MuMTV, called mam [17].

Two out of seven transformed cell lines induced by normal mouse DNA reacted with the antiserum directed against the onc-gene product of A-MuLV. The specificity of the antiserum is evident from the data in Table 3. The antiserum reacted only with cells transformed by A-MuLV, but not with untransformed cell lines infected with Mo- or R-MuLV. The cell lines infected with MuMTV did not react with this antiserum but were stained by the C3Hf mouse antiserum directed against mammary tumor cells. That antiserum did not stain the cell lines transformed by A-MuLV or normal cell DNA.

TABLE 3

Immunofluorescence of Cell Lines with Antisera Directed Against
Onc-Genes of Murine Oncoviruses

Cell Line	Anti A-MuLV-onc	Anti-MuMTV-mam	Normal Mouse Serum
BALB/3T3	-	-	-
+ R-MuMLV	-	-	-
Transf. A-MuMLV	+	-	-
Transf. A-MuMLV-DNA	+	-	-
Transf. normal BALB/c DNA	+ (2/7)	-	-
Moloney sarcoma v	-	-	-
C57BL-A-MuLV-lymphoma	+	-	-
NIH/3T3	-	-	-
+ Mo-MuLV	-	-	-
C3HMT/cl11	-	+	-
Mm5mt/cl	-	+	-
C3HMK/Rij	-	-	-
BMK/A	-	-	-
CrFK	-	-	-
CrFK + MuMTV	-	+	-
FRE	-	+	-

TABLE 4

Effect of Preinfection with Murine Leukemia Virus on
Early Transformation by Normal BALB/c DNA

Recipient Cells	Treatment	Fraction Transformed Cultures at 2 Weeks	Average No. Foci/Dish	Average Transformation Foci x 10^6/μg DNA/Cell
NIH/3T3	BALB/c liver DNA[a]	0/33	0	0
	E. coli DNA	0/33	0	0
	Transfection buffer	0/33	0	0
NIH/3T3-R-MuLV[b]	BALB/c liver DNA	3/3	4	2
	E. coli DNA	0/3	0	0
	Transfection buffer	0/3	0	0
NIH/3T3-Mo-MuLV[c]	BALB/c liver DNA	33/33	18	7
	E. coli DNA	0/33	0	0
	Transfection buffer	0/33	0	0

[a]25 μg.ml^{-1}.

[b]NIH/3T3 infected with Rauscher murine leukemia virus 4 days before transfection.

[c]NIH/3T3-cloned after been productively infected with Moloney murine leukemia virus.

All lines yielded fibrosarcomas on inoculation into nude mice. Except for one line, they also produced tumors when subcutaneously injected into BALB/c or (BALB/c x DBA/2)F1 mice. Tumors appeared within three weeks.

We attempted to increase the transformation rate by treating the recipient cells with DMSO, glycerol or polybrene + hydrocortisone + insuline. Neither compound had an effect. However, preinfection of the cells with a murine leukemia virus resulted in a strong increase in the transformation frequency (Table 4). Foci were detectable within two weeks after one passage. The transformation frequency was as high as that found for DNA isolated from A-MuLV lymphoma cells: 1 focus forming unit per µg DNA. This indicates that approximately 1 pg of DNA must be provided per cell for one focus to appear in a dish seeded with 3×10^5 cells. A linear dose-response relationship was found in this system (Figure 1).

So far, we failed to detect transforming activity in the supernatants of cultures infected with Mo-MuLV and transformed by BALB/c DNA.

DISCUSSION

Since DNA isolated from different tissues of BALB/c mice can transform either kind of 3T3 cells, it seems that transforming genes are present in the germ line of this mouse strain. We are presently investigating, whether DNA from other mouse strains or rodents has similar transforming capacity.

It does not seem likely that the transforming capacity of normal cell DNA is due to some mutagenic action of this substance, since E. coli and calf thymus DNA are ineffective in this system. Integration of specific nucleotide sequences into the host genome must be responsible for neoplastic conversion of the recipient cells. In the experiments with MuLV-infected cells the single-hit kinetics (Figure 1) indicate that incorporation of a single DNA fragment would be sufficient for transformation. It remains to be established whether the same holds for uninfected recipient cells.

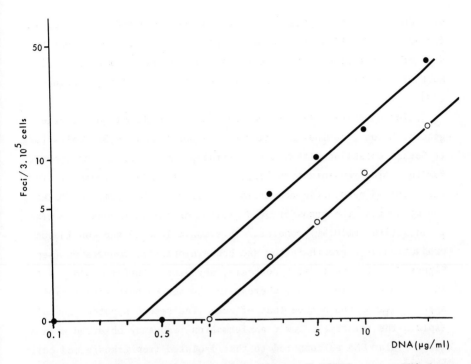

Figure 1. Relationship between dose of normal BALB/c mouse DNA fragments and number of foci of transformed cells in NIH/3T3 cells infected
with Moloney murine leukemia virus, obtained in two separate experiments.

The immunofluorescence data suggest that in 2 out 7 cases the
cellular homologue of the onc-gene of A-MuLV has been transferred.
Probably several other genes in normal cellular DNA have the potential
to transform fibroblasts in vitro. We intend to investigate the cellu-
lar-derived onc-genes of other murine retroviruses in this respect.

It is tempting to assume that these transforming genes in normal
cellular DNA have a function in growth control in the normal cell.
Their expression would be normally regulated in a coordinated manner.
We have hypothesized earlier, that this was achieved by cis-dominant
acting neighbouring regulatory genes [18]. The transfer of the growth
control gene to other sites in the cellular genome would result in
the abrogation of negative control by such regulatory genes. There
is some evidence for such a kind of negative position-dependent control

of endogenous MuMTV [19,20]. Since some rat hepatoma cell lines infected with MuMTV do not produce viral RNA it is concluded that the
site of integration of the exogenous provirus is of importance [21].
Most likely, this is due to negative control by flanking sequences
[20].

Cloned murine cellular sequences which are homologous to the onc-
gene of Moloney murine sarcoma virus cannot transform 3T3 cells [22].
It became established that a retroviral promoter region was needed
for in vitro transformation [23]. As an alternative hypothesis for
the observed neoplastic conversion of 3T3 cells by normal cellular
DNA we suggest the transfer of a growth control gene to a site next
to an active cellular promotor. This would lead to the continuous
production of a growth factor and hence neoplastic conversion (see
Figure 2). In the first hypothesis, any gene-transfer would result
in unregulated expression, whereas in the second only integration at
specific sites would have that effect. The second hypothesis would
explain the relatively low transformation frequency observed with normal cellular DNA as compared to that isolated from transformed cells
[11,12].

Both hypotheses have in common that the transforming action of
normal cellular DNA is due to a change in position of growth-controlling genes. They need not be mutually exclusive: the position effect
can be due to abrogation of negative control by cis-dominant acting
regulatory genes and insertion of the growth-controlling gene next to
active promotor sequences.

The enhancing effect of preinfection with MuLV resembles the co-
carcinogenic effect of MuLV on in vitro transformation of fibroblasts
by chemical carcinogens [24]. The enhancement may be due to the induction of a semi-transformed state of the 3T3 cells by MuLV. We
favor at the moment the alternative hypothesis that MuLV would provide
highly active promotor sequences (Figure 2).

The finding that normal cellular DNA can transform fibroblasts
into cancer cells indicates that the cellular inserts in the genome
of rapidly transforming retroviruses need not be perturbated to be
oncogenic. It supports the hypothesis that tumor induction by nonviral

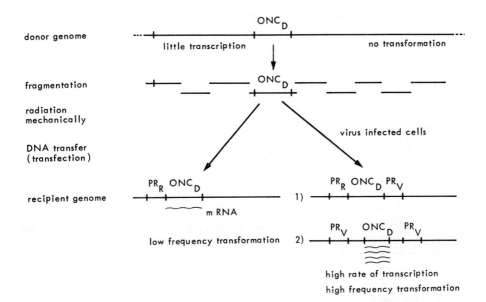

Figure 2. Onc-gene promotion model. Low frequency of transformation occurs when the transforming gene in the donor genome (ONC_D) is fragmented by radiation or mechanically and after transfer to recipient cells has been inserted adjacent to a promotor region (PR_R) in the cellular genome. Insertion of ONC_D in between two promotors (provided by virus - PR_V - or the recipient cell - PR_R) results in a high frequency of transformation.

carcinogens is not due to simple point mutations leading to altered gene products but to genetic changes which result in continuous and enhanced expression of genes controlling cellular proliferation.

We have earlier advanced the hypothesis that radiation carcinogenesis involves the release of DNA fragments from lethally damaged cells and the subsequent uptake of these fragments by another cell which is in either S-phase or in the repair process, resulting in incorporation of growth-controlling genes at sites other than the original one [18]. The findings reported in this paper support this gene transfer-misrepair hypothesis of radiation-carcinogenesis, which may have important implications for estimations of carcinogenic risks at low radiation doses. Presently, these estimations are based on a linear extrapolation model.

If radiation-induction DNA repair is important in terms of carcinogenic risks when compared to normal DNA synthesis, extrapolation on a linear basis does not seem to be warranted as radiation would be required for the induction of donor cells, releasing DNA, as well as the fraction of transformable receptor cells which undergo DNA repair. An equally important consequence of the proposed mechanism of radiation carcinogenesis is that the effects of repeated small radiation doses and those of continuous low dose rate exposure would not accumulate.

Molecular biological technology is becoming available to investigate whether radiation carcinogenesis indeed involves this gene transfer-misrepair mechanism, as has been made more likely by our present findings.

ACKNOWLEDGMENT

This investigation was partially supported by the Koningin Wilhelmina Fonds, The Netherlands Cancer Organization. Skilled technical assistance was given by Mr. R. H. van Leersum, Mr. D. S. Luyt and Mr. M. A. Dubbeld.

REFERENCES

1. Scolnick, E. M., Rands, E., Williams, D. and Parks, W. P., *J. Virol.*, *12*:458-463 (1973).

2. Scolnick, E. M. and Parks, W. P., *J. Virol.*, *13*:1211-1219 (1974).

3. Frankel, A. E. and Fishinger, P. J., *Proc. Nat. Acad. Sci.*, *U.S.A.*, *73*:3705-3709 (1976).

4. Spector, D. H., Varmus, H. E. and Bishop, J. M., *Proc. Nat. Acad. Sci.*, *U.S.A.*, *75*:4102-4106 (1978).

5. Frankel, A. E., Gilbert, J. H., Porzig, K. J., Scolnick, E. M. and Aaronson, S. A., *J. Virol.*, *30*:821-827 (1979).

6. Scolnick, E. M., Howk, R. S., Anisowicz, A., Peebles, P. T.,
    Scher, C. D. and Parks, W. P., *Proc. Nat. Acad. Sci., U.S.A.,*
    *72:*4650-4654 (1975).

7. Roussel, M., Saule, S., Lagrou, C., Rommens, C., Beug, H., Graft,
    T. and Stehelin, D., *Nature, 281:*452-455 (1979).

8. Baltimore, D., Rosenberg, N. and Witte, O. N., *Immunol. Rev.,*
    *48:*3-22 (1979).

9. Stephenson, J. R., Khan, A. S., Van der Ven, W. J. M. and Reynolds,
    F. H. Jr., *J. Natl. Cancer Inst., 63:*1111-1119 (1979).

10. Temin, H. M., The protovirus hypothesis and cancer. In: RNA
    Viruses and Host Genome in Oncogenesis (P. Emmelot and P.
    Bentvelzen, eds.), North-Holland, Amsterdam, 1972, pp. 351-363.

11. Shih, C., Shilo, B., Goldfarb, M. P., Dannenberg, A. and Weinberg,
    R. A., *Proc. Nat. Acad. Sci., U.S.A., 76:*5714-5718 (1979).

12. Cooper, G. M., Okenquist, S. and Silverman, L., *Nature, 284:*418-
    421 (1980).

13. Graham, F. L. and Van der Eb, A. J., *Virology, 52:*456-467 (1973).

14. Westenbrink, F., Koornstra, W., Creemers, P., Brinkhof, J. and
    Bentvelzen, P., *Europ. J. Cancer, 15:*109-121 (1979).

15. Aboud, M., Weiss, O. and Salzberg, S., *Inf. Immun., 13:*1626-1632
    (1976).

16. Witte, O. N., Rosenberg, N. and Baltimore, D., *Proc. Nat. Acad.*
    *Sci., U.S.A., 75:*2488-2492 (1978).

17. Hilgers, J. and Bentvelzen, P., *Adv. Cancer Res., 26:*143-195
    (1978).

18. Van Bekkum, D. W., Mechanisms of radiation carcinogenesis. In:
    Radiation Research, Biomedical, Chemical and Physical Perspectives
    (O. F. Nygaard, H. I. Adler and W. K. Sinclair, eds.), Academic
    Press, New York, 1975, pp. 886-894.

19. Bentvelzen, P., *Biochim. Biophys. Acta, 355:*236-259 (1974).

20. Bentvelzen, P. and Hilgers, J., Murine mammary tumour virus.
    In: Viral Oncology (G. Klein, ed.), Raven Press, New York, 1980,
    pp. 311-355.

21. Ringold, G. M., Shank, P. R., Varmus, H. E., Ring, J. and
    Yamamoto, K. R., *Proc. Nat. Acad. Sci., U.S.A., 76:*665-669 (1979).

22. Oskarsson, M., McClements, W. L., Blair, D. G., Maizel, J. V.
     and Van de Woude, G. F., *Science, 207*:1222-1224 (1980).

23. Van de Woude, G. F., Oskarsson, M., Enquist, L. W., Nomura, S.,
     Sullivan, M. and Fischinger, P. J., *Proc. Nat. Acad. Sci., U.S.A.,
     76*:4464-4468 (1979).

24. Huebner, R. J. and Gilden, R. V., Inherited RNA viral genomes
     (virogenes and oncogenes) in the etiology of cancer. In: RNA
     Viruses and Host Genome in Oncogenesis. (P. Emmelot and P.
     Bentvelzen, eds.), North-Holland, Amsterdam, 1972, pp. 197-219.

INDEX